Praise for Rosetta Taylor-Metz

Taylor-Metz knows that *life happens*. She takes the reader with on her journey to navigate challenges, let go of baggage, and take steps to build the life of her dreams. With anecdotes from her own remarkable life and those of grateful clients, this book reminds us that we're not alone as we figure it all out.

— T. Sticha, MBA, Director of Strategic
Initiatives at Cristo Rey Jesuit High School

It is so easy to find yourself overwhelmed. Rosetta Taylor-Metz takes the approach of a thoughtful friend, with a gentle shake to remind you the best path to peace is to prioritize yourself and your joy. The welcoming and approachable 'joyful practices' prime you to take on the challenging but essential work of finding what is meant for you, even as 'life happens'.

— Erica McKenzie, Legal Administrator,
Boeing

Rosetta Taylor-Metz captures the essence of what it feels like to live in a state of chaos – *and* how to take *real* steps towards a more joyful way of living to get *real* results. You will not only feel validated through this Joy Journey, but gain insight on how to truly change your way of life.

— Marilyn Rose, Writer-Editor, Best Version
Media

This book truly spoke to my soul. As someone with ADHD who's long avoided organization like the plague and constantly added to my plate instead of clearing space, Rosetta's approach felt like a breath of fresh air. She doesn't preach or judge like so many organizing books I've read before. Instead, she meets you where you are—with empathy, grace, and an understanding that life *does* happen, especially for women juggling so much. Her words go far beyond just tidying a home—they offer a way to clear mental and emotional clutter too. For the first time, organizing felt possible—and even empowering.

— DANI, HUMAN RESOURCE MANAGER, BLITT & GAINES

Rosetta Taylor-Metz is the catalyst we all need to jumpstart our journey to a more organized and fulfilling space and life!

— AMELIA BANINI, REGISTERED NURSE PMH-BC, NORTHWESTERN MEMORIAL HOSPITAL

The writing style is engaging and easy to follow, while the writing itself is relatable. Rosetta's perspective on inevitable stress is thought-provoking.

— HAILEY FISHMAN RD, LD REGISTERED DIETITIAN ASCENSION SAINT ALEXIUS

Truly a valuable resource, looking forward to putting into action the "joyful practice" Rosetta recommends.

— AMY ADLER, SENIOR COUNSEL, SHURE INCORPORATED

The Joy Journey

Discover what drives you to live well and fully

Rosetta Taylor-Metz

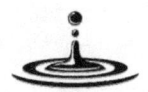

Red Thread Books

Write to **info@redthreadbooks.com** if you are interested in publishing with Red Thread Publishing. Learn more about publications or foreign rights acquisitions of our catalog of books: www.redthreadbooks.com

Paperback ISBN: 979-8-89294-026-9

Ebook ISBN: 979-8-89294-027-6

Cover Design: Red Thread Designs

Contents

DEDICATION

*For my mother, husband and children, who inspire, love and support.
I am blessed to have you all in my heart.* 🤍

Preface

What if you are in survival mode and don't know it? Life is short, and you deserve to live in the moment and not continuously wake up in the past.

What if I told you there are simple ways to focus on you, and joyful moments will appear?

Who would like to feel in control of their lives, free from judgment, anxiety, and obstacles that interfere with our day-to-day existence? Having "control" can be merely an imaginary concept that is the key to sparking a little joy and happiness.

Taking a deep dive into what may be the key to our spark of joy in our journey and how it can be a reality in our day-to-day lives is worth tapping into.

The Joy Journey empowers women (though this is not exclusive to women only) to understand their life motivations and cultivate positive, healthy habits so that they can joyfully live in the moment.

What drives you or how to get there does not have to be a mystery. I will give you the know-how to sort through day-to-day routines to find the driving force of your motivation. This will bring you to action.Think about what you are searching for and what might need to happen to get it done. It should be more than checking it off your list; it should bring joy.

> *"Economics comes in whenever more of one thing means less of another."*
>
> — FRITZ MACHLUP

What is your Why? People live their lives doing what they are "supposed to do." This motivation came from upbringing, past experiences, or observations of others that brought us to where we are today. Understanding the real motivation behind choosing one over the other is what *The Joy Journey* will bring.

> *"We all have to pay a price. You get to choose the price you pay."*
>
> — BOB PROCTOR

Survival mode comes in all shapes and sizes. One day, you wake up exhausted and overwhelmed with multiple kids, a partner, a pet. The impossible schedule to follow and a home filled with stuff. Never mind the career you had. Are you a perfectionist? A control freak? Or do you let everything go except the superficial aspects of life? How did you get here? Aren't you so tired of being out of breath in that constant fight or flight?

We're very good at survival mode and are often entirely unaware that we are in it. You know who I am talking about: the Beverly Goldbergs, obsessive, controlling, perfect PTO volunteer. How about Miranda

Priestly, The Devil Wears Prada, who gives up her personal values only to have control over her business ambitions. Her protege, Andy, finds herself falling into the same trap as her boss. What are you willing to give up to make it up the corporate ladder or to be that perfect mom?

Unfortunately, extra responsibilities do fall on women, such as caring for an elderly parent, raising her children, keeping the home in order, etc., so much so that these responsibilities turn into unhealthy routines. They put you into an autopilot mode that takes the "me" out of the equation, leading to burnout.

Childhood trauma. False belief systems are created because of past experiences. Women need to find ways to push through it. Past choices and circumstances make you who you are.

Growing up the youngest of eleven brothers and sisters was an incredible playground. Positive or negative, it is what made me who I am today. My experiences throughout my life have provided me with finding my true joy which is simply to help others find theirs. Creating Lettuce Organize LLC provided me with the platform to do just this.

I am an extremely empathetic being. I blame it on growing up in chaos. Working with my clients sends triggers throughout my body. My empathy for them on top of my individual experience motivates me to find the best solutions they are looking for. I want you to know you have the power. I am committed to helping you in understanding your life's motivation to cultivate positive, healthy habits.

Each chapter will provide exercises for you to take deep dives into self-discovery and create solutions.

There is a "Think About It" section at the end of each chapter. Use these reflections as affirmations of what you have learned and create your own mindful *intentions* along the way.

∽

THINK ABOUT IT...

I want to have a better understanding of who I am.

I want to understand why I am doing certain things.

I want to live joyfully in the now.

MY INTENTIONS...

I intend to journal my feelings before I go to sleep.

CHAPTER 1

LIFE HAPPENS

WHEN LIFE HAPPENS

"Do you see me cry without tears
Have you been hearing my silent scream
Are my wounds invisible to you
Can you not taste my pain
Are you numb to my suffering

This is not how it should be
A life I live that is not my own
I am invisible to the world and yet I am of the world
How long will my struggle continue"

— MIXO MALEPFANE

What's your story? We will explore a few concepts to help you with the overwhelmingness of "Life Happens." I want you to realize you are not alone. Make a few simple adjustments to help you find a little calm; this will change your mindset from "I can't do this!" to "I got this!"

There's always a story. You heard the expression "...has a lot of baggage" You can be a glass-half-full or, you can be a glass-half-empty. Either you have the answer to everything or are too exhausted to even try. What's the point? Everyone has baggage; this "baggage" is what makes our story. It does not define us; our experiences provide opportunities to grow.

Life can be complex and beautiful. Understanding yourself and having or not having control over your circumstances is difficult to accept. When your world is unraveling or spinning out of control, you feel over-whelmed, distraught, and confused. It's natural to try to control every-thing, and hang on so hard that when the rope breaks, you fly into a chaotic state. You find yourself in this darkness, holding on to an unex-pected reality.

Stress creeps into everyone's lives through every experience. How each experience or interaction is handled can significantly impact the stress level. Over time, you begin to feel powerless. My friend was notorious for this in making New Year's diet resolutions. Starting out strong, using an app and starving herself until the obvious FAIL crept in. Back to old habits, shaming herself with every bite. It doesn't need to be this way.

Think about life-changing events that have happened to you. Loss can be paralyzing, like losing a child or receiving so much rejection in your life, you feel powerless. Learning to distract from what has happened and not taking in any of the emotions you should be processing is your go-to solution. Finding the "joy" in all the negatives and pretty much-ignoring reality is not how to go about it either. This will spin you off into survival mode. Making sure you continue "being busy" instead of taking inventory of yourself. I get it. I would rather keep this to myself as nobody would understand what I am going through. When working with my clients, I have asked: *What do you do when you spin out of control? What have you been doing to cope? Do you isolate?*

As a Professional Organizer, I help people sort through their dreams, regrets, happiness, and reality; offer some peace of mind. Inside the office or at home, I strategize with my clients to help them develop better habits, increase their self-esteem, and find that little piece of joy. "Life Happens" as you can hear it in this common conversation I had with Susie (made-up name, but real person).

Susie says,

> Hi, thank you for coming. I was going to clean up before you got here, but the cat threw up, and I had to get my daughter to daycare and my son to the bus stop.

> > It's nice to meet you. No worries. How about you walk me through the areas in the home that are making you crazy.

As Susie gulps her mega-size iced coffee with a cup of sugar, we walk.

> Sure, this is the living room, and we just dump our coats here and watch out—don't trip on the toys there. Here is the dining room, but we don't use it, as it is our dumping ground for the mail and stuff. I have no idea what is on or under the table. Why don't I show you the kitchen? Um, well, breakfast is still out, as this morning was kind of crazy, (melting ice dripping from the counter to the floor) and we just didn't get a chance to clean up from dinner last night. And as you can see, we have a problem with boxes. I am organized, and I have never been like this; it's just that a lot is going on, and I don't know where to begin. I am sorry it's like this.

> > Let's sit down and talk. I understand that life happens, and it's okay. You are not alone, and you don't need to apologize. I am here to help, and we will figure this out together.

It's okay to ask for help. When resolutions, plans, and projects fall apart, the entire body feels the stress. When you put unnecessary imaginary pressure on yourself, self-doubt and negative thoughts seep in. When loss is not dealt with or processed, isolation can become a haven.

We have all had that experience when you wake up and it's 1:30 am. The mind is racing, and your thoughts are everywhere but at rest. In just a few sleep-deprived hours, you will be getting your kids ready for school, your dog walked and fed, and yourself ready for work.

Alarm sounds! Grab clothes off the dusty treadmill in your bedroom, take a shower, and don't forget your make-up for the road. Open the doors to your kids' rooms, yell to them to get ready for school. Take the dog out on a quick morning walk before you leave.

"You are late. Let's go!" You got to get breakfast in the kitchen, no-time; grab Pop-Tarts for the kids to eat in the car or at the bus stop. Don't lie, you know you are also eating the blueberry Pop-Tart as you run out the door. You are already exhausted before the day has even begun.

Life happens. Your baggage is showing! Time to acknowledge the stress you are having doesn't feel good. Reduce this stress. What is stopping you? How do you begin to do anything for yourself when you do not have the time?

It can be a problem of overcommitting. It is important to learn when to say no without feeling guilty. How often are you overwhelmed with too much work because you feel nobody can do it except you? Find ways to give it to others to free up more time for yourself. Why do you feel it is your responsibility to solve everyone else's problems? Time to learn how to set clear boundaries.

DO IT NOW! NOW IS THE TIME

Throughout this book, I have created "Joyful Practice" exercises to allow readers to apply what was taught in the chapter or challenge themselves.

JOYFUL PRACTICE

Here is a list to get you started on getting back to you. Choose one action from the list and keep it simple.

1. Prioritize fewer high impact activities; add to your low impact activities. Habit Stack; you can listen to audio-books while running or while driving. Remove resistance - visualize how you want to feel.
2. Create a routine. This is helpful; it can remove the anxiety of not knowing what's next or provide the comfort of preparing yourself. The routine should be flexible but have enough structure to help you get it done. If you are an early riser, try to get up earlier. It could be getting up 30 minutes earlier and enjoying your favorite morning drink in your favorite cozy place in your home (your happy spot). And finally meditate – use an app or close your eyes and clear your mind for whatever lies ahead of you.
3. Get Organized. Start putting your tasks on a calendar.
4. Create obtainable goals. Be sure there is a plan or steps for achieving them.
5. Put "me time" into your schedule. Monday at 8 am – have a cup of coffee in a sunny room, walk through the forest preserve, or read a book.
6. Write a to-do list daily (manually, on your phone or computer).
7. Boost your mood. Listen to music, dance, or laugh.
8. Journal – have a journal (notebook), write something wonderful about yourself or a grateful moment every night before you sleep.
9. Just BREATHE. Take a moment for yourself before you get up in the morning, do some deep breathing and some positive thoughts before starting your day.
10. Continue to do one simple task for yourself for at least 18 days so that it has a chance to become a habit.

Science tells us that for a habit to form, it must be repeated. Creating new behavior may take two to six months, depending on the person. It doesn't mean you can only do one thing at a time. Also, don't let these stats overwhelm you. Find the one joyful activity and just do it. The joy or calm it brings will be your motive to stick with it.

Life happens! Don't allow it to take over so you lose touch with your dreams and reality. Social media is just one outlet you may choose to create the mind-set you wish to have. "Here's a photo of my perfect husband and my perfect kids." Hmm, how many likes? You are posting on Social Media about what was accomplished just for the gratification of everyone liking the post. A love for posting develops, and you do it often. Take a step back and enjoy the moment without documenting it.

Your social media can show you what you are going through. Are you posting to reassure yourself that you are the perfect parent or have the ideal job? Are you looking for approval?

> *"Let go of the approval of others, especially those who are not the most important people in your life."*
>
> — DAILY MOTIVATION

Another outlet is your children's well-being. This baggage you are carrying is influencing how you raise your children. It can feel like they are missing something if they don't take that class or play that sport. "Keeping up with the Joneses," FOMO "Fear of Missing Out." These are real. If the other kids are playing tennis, playing in the traveling league, taking piano, etc., shouldn't yours?

You want your children to have the best available experiences and opportunities. It's natural to compare yourself to other parents doing similar activities for their children. You can get into this cycle unconsciously and book every minute into an activity.

Life happens; everyone is over-scheduled. It is essential to take a step back and see if all of you are getting the most out of your time. Look to see if your children are positively interacting with other kids. Does excitement drive them to get ready? Or are you constantly after them to practice, get ready for their planned activities?

Take inventory of how many tantrums occur or if they procrastinate every time they are on to their next activity. Be mindful of how much is too much and what they seem to excel in. How are their schedules affecting you?

You don't have to have kids to also fall into this trap. FOMO can apply to you and your personal life. Do you participate in networking activities only because your colleagues are doing them? Are you the person who gets talked into joining every church and committee group, or is in charge of the next project at work? Are you the caregiver to your parent, taking on all the responsibilities without asking for help? Life happens and you are in the midst of doing too much and now navigating through these overscheduled days.

It is great to be driven to get things done. However, no matter how organized and driven you might be, clearly understanding why and how you are doing what you do helps unravel your life's motivation.

JOYFUL PRACTICE

Write your thoughts or feelings around the following questions and keep them nearby while navigating through this book.

1. Are you taking time for yourself?
2. Are you working towards your hopes and dreams?
3. Are you allowing your children to take time for themselves?
4. Is everything important to you organized, or just the busy schedules?
5. What habits or patterns do you currently have that contribute to stress or your aspirations?
6. What are your goals and dreams?

∾

THINK ABOUT IT...

I want to start new, simple habits like journaling.

I want to make time for myself.

I will not isolate myself.

MY INTENTIONS...

I intend to do one thing this week for myself.

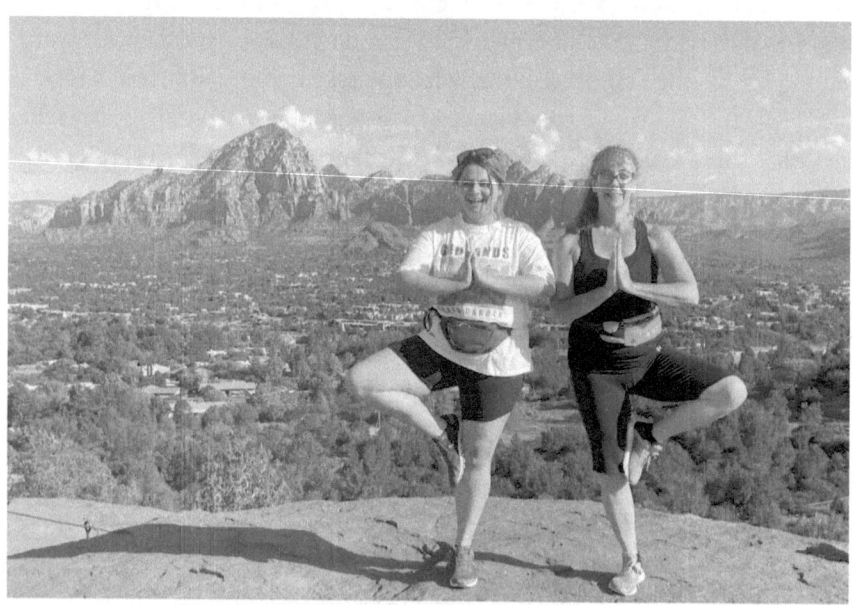

Chapter 2

See and Feel What You Want

This chapter will get you to where you want to go. Let's start visualizing what you want your day to look and feel like. Maslow's Hierarchy of Needs is sometimes used to gain an understanding of certain areas of our lives that need immediate attention. If that attention is not taken, then moving on to other areas in your life will be difficult.

Let me introduce you to "The Seven Readjustment Steps," an evaluation tool I created that helps identify areas in your life that you can improve. Understanding the hierarchy of needs and using the adjustment steps will help visualize how you want your day to be.

Joyful Practice

Sit in a comfortable position on a chair or the floor. Close your eyes. Take a deep breath through your nose slowly (count 1, 2, 3, 4), hold your breath (count 1, 2, 3, 4) and slowly exhale through your nose (count 1, 2, 3, 4), hold your breath (count 1, 2, 3, 4). Repeat.

Visualize yourself in your happy place whether in the woods, on the water, or skiing down a mountain. Maybe it's as simple as sitting quietly some-

where in your home. Breathe normally, focus on the pleasure this place brings you.

Focus on this happy spark. Feel this sensation and remember it. Let this be the feeling you want your day to feel like.

Take one more deep breath, and slowly open your eyes.

Now, let's get to work!

Let's Consider Maslow's Hierarchy of Needs

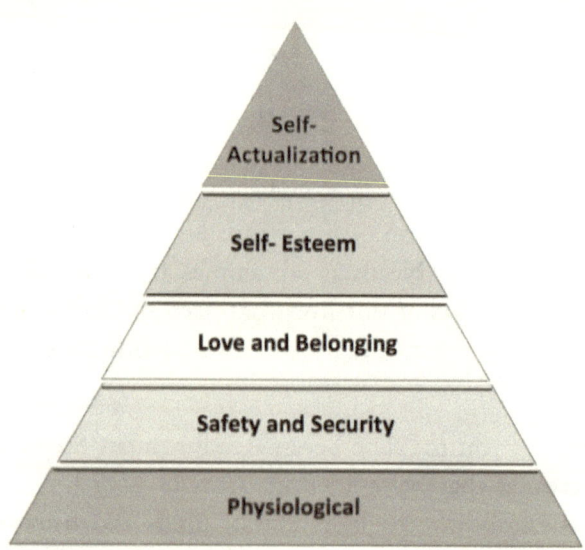

Psychologist Abraham Maslow created the Hierarchy of Needs. Human beings are motivated by a hierarchy of needs. Needs are organized in a hierarchy of prepotency in which more basic needs must be more or less met (rather than all or none) before higher needs. The order of needs is not rigid but instead may be flexible based on external circumstances or individual differences. Most behavior is multi-motivated, that is simultaneously determined by more than one basic need. Self-actualization is considered a Growth Need. Motivation increases here as the desire to improve yourself.

"It is quite true that man lives by bread alone — when there is no bread. But what happens to man's desires when there is plenty of bread and when his belly is chronically filled?

At once, other (and "higher") needs emerge, and these, rather than physiological hunger, dominate the organism. And when these, in turn are satisfied, again new (and still "higher") needs emerge, and so on. This is what it means by saying that the basic human needs are organized into a hierarchy of relative prepotency" (Maslow, 1943, p. 375).

DEFICIENCY NEEDS

1. Physiological Needs - Food, Water, Shelter; Basic Human Needs
2. Safety Needs - Security and Stability Needs
3. Love and Belonging Needs - Love and Community
4. Esteem Needs - Self-Esteem and Recognition from Others

GROWTH NEED

1. Self-Actualization Need

Maslow's Hierarchy of Needs - Simply Psychology.

Maslow's Hierarchy Of Needs (A Complete Guide) | OptimistMinds.

JOYFUL PRACTICE

Where Are You on Maslow's Hierarchy of Needs? Write down your answers to the questions at each level and see if you find patterns of behavior or ways to improve your day-to-day bringing more joy.

Let's simplify this and apply it to how you are living your life. Let's look at the bottom of the triangle. **Physiological Needs** should be the first to be met.

How are you taking care of yourself? Are you eating healthy, are you hydrated, are you able to support yourself or are you dependent on someone else, and are you responsible for others?

It's important to take care of yourself. If you are dependent on others in various areas, you will need to work on finding additional ways to be more independent. Also, if you are responsible for taking care of others, can you get help? Are you motivated to do this or is something holding you back?

Next, look at your **Safety Needs**.

Do you feel safe where you are living, do you feel safe with who you are living with, and how stable is your day-to-day life?

There should be additional check-ins on how you are feeling. If you are not living in a safe area, finding the motivation to do so will be important. Also, connecting self-care here, it is ok to ask for help, especially if you are in an unhealthy or dangerous relationship or situation. Energy spent here will bring you closer to feeling more joy in your journey. You are worth it.

Love and Belonging Needs are the third level in the triangle.

Are you in a healthy relationship, do you engage with others or isolate yourself, and do you have a community in your daily life?

It is better for our health to have love in our lives. Love for others, having a community to support you, finding commonalities that you can relate to, and having a desire to give back to your community are all good things.

Let's look at **Esteem Needs** and how they may affect us in our daily lives.

Do you feel good about yourself? Do you feel others respect you? Are you dependent on what others tell you, do you surround yourself with like-minded people, and are you with positive or negative people?

Checking in on how you feel when you are with certain people can be a healthy exercise. The people you choose to engage with can have a strong effect on how you feel about yourself and others. It's a good practice to check in with your feelings (anxious, angry, etc.) and try to understand why you feel this way. Many times, it is who you are with that has that negative or positive effect on how you feel. If it's too much work, then maybe spend less time with them. Find what can motivate you to embrace like-minded people or re-evaluate how you feel about who you are with.

Finally, you are at the top of the triangle: **Self-Actualization Needs**.

Are you working towards your full potential? Do you know what is driving you, what is stopping you from achieving your goals, and do you recognize patterns in your life that keep holding you back?

This is a good step to check in on your growth as a human being. You are progressing to who you want to be. Where you are on your journey should show up here. How can you find ways to continue moving yourself forward? Education, new jobs, new habits, and new hobbies are among many amazing activities to bring joy to your journey.

"Insanity is doing the same thing over and over and expecting different results."

Seven Readjustment Steps

It can be overwhelming to figure out how to get and stay organized. There are ways to reduce the stress you may be feeling. Start by becoming aware of the areas in your life you'd like to improve. The Seven Readjustment Steps help you evaluate your current situation and rethink your next steps with care to help develop better solutions. It's all about creating a system that works for you and is simple to maintain/readjust when necessary.

1. *Review* Various Areas of Your Life—Categories can include, but are not limited to: Home, Work, Family, Finances, Personal Growth/Spirituality, Health, Etc.

2. *Determine Priorities—Determine which* aspects of your life are most relevant. Review your list in Step 1. Identify and narrow your list to what is most significant to your daily life.
3. *Identify Problems—*What types of issues/challenges continuously show up?
4. *Resolve Problems—*What options do you have? What is in your control? What support systems are you working with?
5. *Redesign Processes* In Your Life—This will become your new habit. Visualize what your life might look like if you did things differently. Doing just one simple task for yourself each day can make a difference.
6. *Prioritize—*Think about what's most important to you.
7. *Maintenance—*Think about the systems you have in place. Are they helping you maintain the processes you have created in Step 5? Tweak whatever is not working as you go.

JOYFUL PRACTICE

This exercise can be found in **Chapter Eleven** and will explore each Readjustment Step more deeply. Go ahead and go through the exercise while it's fresh in your mind. If not, go back to it later.

How did it go? Did you add at least one new redesign (habit)? You can always talk with someone you trust to help you narrow down your life categories. Isolating is one of my go-to strategies when I do not think I need help. However when I do finally engage, I come to the realization that I am not alone.

I wish I had this tool or information when I was younger to reevaluate my schedule and learn how to prioritize what is important. Below, I share a story about "Emily," named change to protect the innocent.

> *Emily found herself volunteering or starting various committees in her community, continuously starting or joining multiple networking groups, committing to an overwhelming number of projects at work. Eventually, she found herself missing an imperative meeting at work and almost losing her job.*

Emily spun out-of-control. Instead of reviewing what she was spending her time on and reevaluating her priorities, she decided she would begin saying no from now on, no matter what. Finding that she had no time to do things like hang out with friends or family, she began saying "No" to family events and to friends and continued to say "Yes" to everything else.

Emily's friends and family started to get upset with her because she would NOT say "Yes" to any of them. Their reaction began to make Emily feel mad, and sad. She did not have time for herself. Emily began to isolate herself from the ones she loved but continued to be busy with all her other commitments.

*Until Emily finally realized she wasn't happy. She wanted **the joy back into her life.** She worked with me to reassess what she was spending her time on and was able to reprioritize. Finally, she made herself a priority and found herself enjoying time with her friends and family once again. She got back **the joy in her journey.***

It is not a selfish act to take care of you! Take the time to see what you are doing.

THINK ABOUT IT...

I want to take time for me.

I want less stress.

I know it is not selfish to focus on me.

MY INTENTIONS...

I intend to focus on one area of my life that I want to improve.

CHAPTER 3

CREATE A LIVABLE PLAN

"She,
In the dark,
Found light
Brighter than many ever see.

And now the world receives
From her dower:
The message of the strength
Of inner power."

— LANGSTON
HUGHES

Through the Joyful Exercises, you will empower yourself to understand your life's motivation (purpose) and cultivate positive, healthy habits to live in the moment joyfully.

A new concept, The Seven Wastes, is introduced. You will apply it to the Seven Readjustment Steps from the last chapter to begin creating the Livable Plan^{SM}. A Livable Plan is the framework to build, cultivate, to transform your daily life. Think of it as your toolbox. As you learn how to use the concepts (tools) throughout this book, you can come back and dig into your toolbox (Livable Plan).

These tools and techniques are here to support you in your journey.

I was fortunate to live in a neighborhood filled with other families with children the same age as mine. When my children were very young and not yet in school, I loved being outdoors no matter what the weather was. We played in the backyard, out front, and at the nearby parks. I would play fun learning games with them. I pictured myself homeschooling my children.

I would open our garage door and organize the toys so they could easily pull them in and out. The neighborhood kids would come by at different times and play all day. I learned about my neighbor's kids' various activities when talking with the moms. I started to second guess what I was doing with my kids and began to compare it with what they were doing with theirs. Uh oh, is this where it starts?

Let's think about the "unnecessary" in our everyday lives—the wasteland of the daily chaos you surround yourself in, the overscheduling and madness you create. How can you reduce this waste?

THE SEVEN WASTES

"The seven "wastes" ("muda" in Japanese), first formulated by Toyota engineer Shigeo Shingo, are the waste of superfluous inventory of raw material and finished goods.

- The waste of overproduction (producing more than what is needed now).

- The waste of over-processing (processing or making parts beyond the standard expected by customer).
- The waste of transportation (unnecessary movement of people and goods inside the system).
- The waste of motion (mechanizing or automating before improving the method).
- The waste of waiting (inactive working periods due to job queues).
- And the waste of making defective products (reworking to fix avoidable defects in products and processes)."

Lean manufacturing - Wikipedia.

Jonathan Law, ed. (2009), *A Dictionary of Business and Management*, Oxford University Press.

It is a good practice to re-evaluate what you do daily and find the tasks or areas you spend time on that do not serve you well. "The Seven Wastes" are listed below to help us dig deeper into our self-evaluation. A great way to remember our waste list is: you want **A COSIER** Life.

Activity – What can you improve, eliminate, or redesign?
Conveyance – How are you getting there?
Obstruction – What is stopping you?
Shortcoming – What appears to be broken in your everyday life? How is your Quality of Life? What are your defects?
Irrelevant – Are you overthinking it?
Excess – Are you doing too much? Does it bring value?
Reserve – What do you have or need to get you there?

JOYFUL PRACTICE

This Joyful Practice exercise can be found in **Chapter Eleven** and will help you be more specific and accountable to what you set out to do (your new habit). Use your answers from the Seven Adjustment Steps Grid in Chapter Two to re-evaluate your answers with each of the Seven Wastes.

"The most dangerous kind of waste is the waste we don't recognize."

— SHIGEO SHINGO

What common threads have you found after this Joyful Practice exercise using the Seven Readjustment Steps and the Seven Wastes? Below are some common threads from our examples. Do any of these resonate with you?

- Resources
- Fear
- Commitment
- Self Esteem
- Time

Look at Maslow's Hierarchy of Needs as well. It's clear that similar common threads are found. Remember it's when you have met all or most of our Physiological Needs, such as food, water, and shelter, that we can move to the other Needs. Once the first four sets of Needs have been met, you can move toward Self-Actualization Growth Needs.

Our lower-level needs often interrupt our progress, creating fluctuations throughout your life journey. This is why going through these Joyful Practice exercises help you sort through what may be holding you back.

A livable plan is not final. It's a living document and should change as you grow through your life. This means that those moments of JOY can come and go. Finding the best solution is what you are working towards to keep you going.

Diving deeper into the power of habits and how to create them will help you find and sustain your happy moments in time. Creating habits should be simple.

Habits are subconscious behaviors; they're ingrained in your brain. You are triggered by a cue that brings you to the actual behavior, which most likely was conditioned as a reward of some sort to keep you going.

Though not all rewards may always be in our best interest. *An example of this can be "stress eating". When something triggers you in a negative way, you begin to eat all the potato chips, or all the candy bars - that makes you feel good in the moment, in the long run you know it's a bad choice.*

Our habits can have a huge impact on our daily lives. Often programmed (unconscious habits) to do what you do daily, weekly, etc. When you are programmed to complete positive habits, you usually achieve what was set out to do or mentally feel good about what is getting done. It is a win as long as these positive habits are revisited from time to time to ensure the habit still serves us. Circumstances change, and our goals and objectives along the way do also. When this happens, rest assured your habits can change for the better.

A simple example of being programmed can be the following:

Negative Talk is something you do without even thinking about it. I saw this while working with a client to help get her kitchen organized. I noticed that she would pick up an item, such as a crock pot, and find it dirty when she took it out and mumbled to herself, *"How disgusting am I to put this away dirty"* or we would come across a baking pan ,*"I suck at baking, not sure why I even have these."* These comments continued throughout our work together. I asked her to journal every night for at least two weeks, write down at least one compliment about herself, and increase the number of positive comments as time passed.

A few weeks later working with her in another room in her home, she had almost stopped saying bad things about herself. All because of the way she reflected about herself. This made a huge difference in how she later felt. She was acting in a new, positive manner. This negative talk was a habit she created for herself without even recognizing it.

Coming up we will explore the power of habits and learn practical tips for creating positive habits that can improve your life.

Here's how to understand the Habit Loop. The habit loop is a cycle that involves three key components: the cue, the routine, and the reward. The cues you get are the triggers that initiate the habit. The behavior itself becomes routine, and the reward is the positive outcome that reinforces the habit.

The illustration below represents the habit loop, which consists of three parts:

1. **Cue:** The trigger that initiates the habit.
2. **Routine:** The behavior or action that follows the cue.
3. **Reward:** The positive feelings that reinforce the habit.

Over time, this habit loop becomes automatic, and the person may not even consciously think about it. Understanding and manipulating the habit loop's different components makes it possible to create or change habits.

Identifying the **cue, routine**, and **reward** is important when deciding to create a new habit. Another example can be to create a habit of going for a walk every day; you might use the cue of putting on your gym shoes; the routine would be walking for 30 minutes, and the reward is feeling energized and proud.

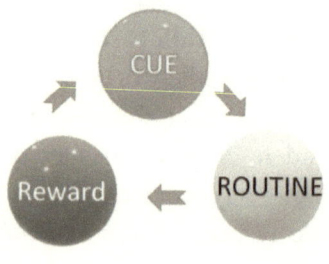

TECHNIQUES FOR CREATING HABITS

1. KISS (Keep it short & simple)
2. Be consistent.
3. Enjoy what you are doing.
4. Find positive ways to encourage yourself to continue.
5. Try to Habit Stack. Brush your teeth before bed; you might add a new habit of doing a quick meditation before brushing.
6. Track your progress.

Understand the habit loop and use the six techniques stated on the previous page. Keep it **simple**, start out small, be **consistent, enjoy** what you are doing, find **positive** vibes when doing it, try **habit stacking**, and finally, **track** your progress. All of these can help you create habits that stick and make your joy journey easier and more enjoyable.

Habit Stacking

Habit Stacking is stacking a new habit onto an existing one. Here's how the habit-stacking process works:

1. Choose an existing habit: *Morning Cup of Coffee*
2. Choose a new habit to stack: *Mindful Meditation*
3. Identify a trigger: *Finishing the coffee*
4. Stack the new habit: *Meditate*

Stacking the new habit onto an existing one; over time, this new habit can become automatic, just like the existing habit. Habit stacking is a powerful tool for creating new habits that stick.

Break a bad habit for a new healthy habit through the creation of a PACT Goal. Let's go back to our example in the "Seven Readjustment Steps" and use the focus on:

- Myself
- Commit to having a specified amount of time for only me
- Get up one hour earlier each morning and meditate.

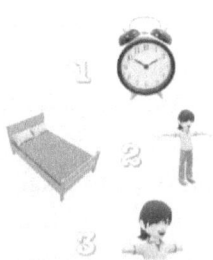

The bad habits illustrated here include not providing time for yourself, sleeping in, and rushing out every morning without any intention for the day.

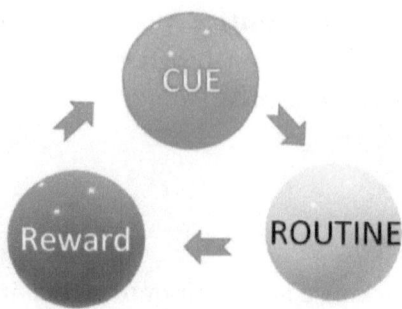

Cue: Alarm - rushing up and out of the house in the morning
Routine: Do this almost every morning
Reward: Extra sleep - hitting the alarm to snooze

You want to commit to a regular meditation schedule in the morning. Your **CUE** is the alarm and rushing out of the house mindlessly with no intention for the day; The **ROUTINE** is every morning and your **REWARD** is hitting the snooze button and getting extra sleep. You want to change this bad habit and apply it to the Joyful Practice below.

Now that we are clear on what we want to change or improve in your daily life from the example above, let's discuss goal-setting tools we want to use.

First, let me share a story about Warren Buffet. This story helps to explain further the importance of prioritizing.

THE STORY OF MIKE FLINT

Mike Flint was Warren Buffett's personal airplane pilot for ten years. (Flint has also flown four US Presidents, so I think you can safely say he is good at his job.) According to Flint, he was talking about his career priorities with Buffett when his boss asked the pilot to go through a three-step exercise.

HERE'S HOW IT WORKS:

STEP 1: Buffett started by asking Flint to write down his top twenty-five career goals. So, Flint took some time to write them down.

> Note: *You could also complete this exercise with goals in smaller chunks. For example, write down the top ten things you want to accomplish this week.*

STEP 2: Then, Buffett asked Flint to review his list and circle his top five goals. Again, Flint took some time, made his way through the list, and eventually decided on his five most important goals.

> Note: *Now you do the same. Choose five out of your ten things you want to accomplish this week.*

STEP 3: At this point, Flint had two lists. The five items he had circled were List A, and the twenty items he had not circled were List B.

Flint confirmed that he would start working on his top five goals right away. And that's when Buffett asked him about the second list, *"And what about the ones you didn't circle?"*

Flint replied, *"Well, the top five are my primary focus, but the other twenty come in a close second. They are still important, so I'll work on those intermittently as I see fit. They are not as urgent, but I still plan to give them a dedicated effort."*

To which Buffett replied, *"No. You've got it wrong, Mike. Everything you didn't circle just became your Avoid-At-All-Cost list. No matter what, these things get no attention from you until you've succeeded with your top five."*

> Warren Buffett's "2 List" Strategy: How to Maximize Your Focus
> —Written by James Clear.

Understanding where you are currently in your struggles, wins, finances, etc., helps prepare you to decide where you want to be. When setting goals, consider your vision for the present day, a week, month... or a year from now.

PACT GOALS

PACT, which stands for **P**urposeful, **A**ctionable, **C**ontinuous, and **T**rackable, is a straightforward yet strong framework we'll explore here.

> **Purposeful:** These goals are deliberately intended to accomplish your goal. These accomplishments relate to your overall plan.
> **Actionable:** The goal or plan is ready to execute.
> **Continuous:** The action of these goals is timeless and can be maintained easily.
> **Trackable:** Tracking results will keep you accountable and bring you back to continuous improvements.

Using the work in the previous Joyful Exercises will help you tighten up your **PACT** Goals.

Before you begin to create a PACT goal, revisiting habits is a good idea. The upcoming Healthy Exercise will combine habits and your PACT goal to bring peace of mind into your daily routines.

Changing a bad habit into a good one using the PACT Goal method.

> **Purposeful:** Using mindfulness, these goals are deliberately intended to accomplish what you set out to do.
> *You will create a new morning routine to ultimately provide stress reduction, feel healthier, and have an intention for your day.*
> **Actionable:** The goal or plan is ready to go.
> *Get up 30 minutes earlier each day, set a new sound on your alarm, and do not hit the snooze button. Find a quiet spot and meditate with a positive intention for each day.*
> **Continuous:** The action of these goals is timeless and can

improve each time. *Find another time to meditate if you accidentally oversleep; maybe take time and meditate at lunch. Return to your new routine the following morning.*
Trackable: Tracking results will keep you accountable and bring you back to continuous improvements as stated above. Keep *track of how many days you are consistent with your new routine. Also, remember to journal how you feel each night before bed.*

New Cue: The new alarm sound gets you up 30 minutes earlier.

Routine: Do this almost every morning.

Reward:Reduced stress, more calmness, and clear positive intentions for the day!

Joyful Practice

Your turn. This exercise can be found in ***Chapter Eleven*** and will guide you into creating your own PACT goal along with your new habit.

This broad exercise of taking one of your top five from your "Seven Readjustment Steps" and applying it to a PACT Goal shows how you can begin to form newer, healthier habits. These new habits can change your life, keep you on track to accomplishing more than you could imagine, and feel those sparks of joy as you move forward.

We now have many tools in your toolbox. As we progress through the Joy Journey, we will add to the Livable Plan. Remember to use what works for you.

∿

THINK ABOUT IT...

I want to be accountable for what I say I am going to do.

I want to be aware of my actions.

I want to understand what is holding me back.

MY INTENTIONS...

I intend to create reachable goals,

Chapter 4

Focus on You

"She sat at the back and they said she was shy,
She led from the front and they hated her pride,
They asked her advice and then questioned her guidance,
They branded her loud, then were shocked by her silence,

But one day she asked what was best for herself,
Instead of trying to please everyone else,
She told them she felt she was never enough,
She was either too little or far too much,
Too loud or too quiet, too fierce or too weak,
Too wise or too foolish, too bold or too meek,

Then she found a small clearing surrounded by firs,
And she stopped... and she heard what the trees said to her,
And she sat there for hours not wanting to leave,
For the forest said nothing, it just let her breathe."

— Becky Helmsley

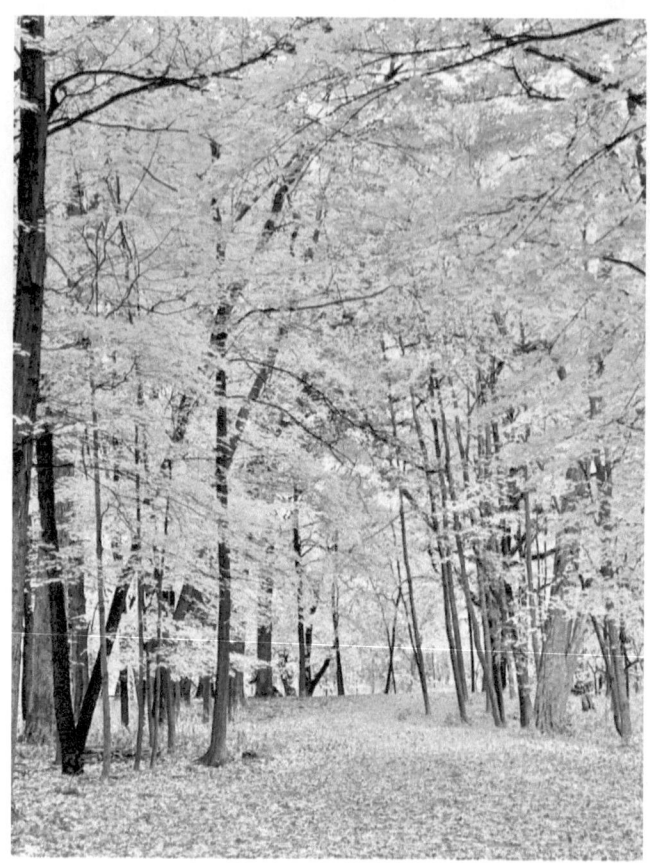

How do you feel when you read this poem? Does any of it resonate with you? What can you identify with? I chose this poem in particular because I want you to search deep into your feelings and understand that it is okay to be the center of attention, loud or quiet. It is alright for you to focus on yourself and be who you are.

Let's focus on you. I will discuss the benefits and how important it is to take care of yourself for your growth, health, and happiness. I will introduce concepts like Grounding and Breathing Techniques to calm your nervous system. I will also cover Al-Anon's 12-Step Program and how these steps can help anyone learn how to focus on themselves and thrive.

The power of focusing on yourself can be a valuable way to improve your daily life. It's easy to lose touch with what you want and need while flying through life. Hours can be spent keeping up with work, and meaningless tasks.

"If you want something done, ask a busy person."

— BENJAMIN FRANKLIN

Busy, getting things done without understanding why you are so busy. I was that busy person, but was I doing things that were essential or important to me and my family? I found that when I put the focus on others and not me, anything I needed never happened —resulting in additional stress, burnout, and being plain ol' tired. Let's explore the importance of putting the focus back on you and what it can bring to your life.

Taking care of you should be a priority, and finding what works through meditation, exercise, or journaling can help. Think about new hobbies or interests and try those on. Take the time to prioritize your health. Below are simple techniques for putting this focus on you.

Self-awareness: Take time to journal your thoughts and emotions. This will help you get to know yourself better. Journaling also helps you be more mindful of how you are feeling and how you want to feel. This habit will keep you on track to be more intentional in your decisions and actions.

Improve your mental health: It is important to have trusted friends and family or even a therapist when you are feeling alone, isolated, or anxious. Having the right support system in place will help you feel secure and confident. Make your mental health a priority. You are worth it!

Find that creativity: Think about things you can do that are creative. Take time out to find this side of you. Draw, paint, dance, etc., and organically, new ideas and perspectives will be born.

Increase your resilience: When you start to know how to handle what comes your way, it will make you a stronger person. Facing into the setbacks that may get thrown your way, having resilience will give you the ability to cope in a healthy and calmer manner.

Relationships Improve: You might find that your relationships with your partner, children, friends start to improve. When you are taking care of yourself, you will be better equipped to show up fully in all of your relationships.

Now that we see the benefits of focusing on ourselves, I would like to show you how we can incorporate this focus into our daily lives.

Joyful Practice

Use this exercise to get in the habit of focusing on yourself. Get a piece of paper or use your computer or phone calendar to schedule yourself to work on the list below. Try at least one of these items listed and gradually add more. See how you feel after doing them.

Set blocked time: Schedule time officially for yourself. Do this on your phone or computer or use a physical calendar on your refrigerator or desk. Set an alarm so you don't forget. Examples can be to get up early in the morning before anyone else is up, or it can be a simple 10-minute break where you can be alone. Use this time to breathe, meditate, or journal. It is important to dedicate this time on a daily basis. As you go along, try to increase the time by at least five minutes. Try a new hobby or interest.

Get physical: Schedule time officially for yourself to engage in a form of exercise that you enjoy. Tennis, running, walking, dancing, yoga, Pilates—anything to get your heart rate moving. Find the one activity that speaks to you and commit to it.

Love yourself: *Treat yourself as you would a friend or family member you enjoy being with. Self-compassion goes a long way in how you feel. Start being as kind to yourself as you are to others.*

Sleep: *Sleep is a good thing! One way to start getting enough sleep is to create a sleep schedule and stick to it. It is so important to prioritize your sleep. Having a good night's sleep is essential for your overall well-being, and this will improve mood, memory, and overall health.*

Journaling: *Schedule time to Journal. Set an alarm if needed. Taking the time to be mindful of what you are grateful for and acknowledging it. Say it out loud! Write it down and see how this will make you feel. When you begin to focus on what you have and not on what you don't have (I wish I had a nicer car like my neighbor, I wish I could travel to another country, etc.), it will change your brain's thought process by focusing on what you achieved, or you have instead of what you wish you had. This does not mean that you cannot push yourself to obtain things you want; it means to appreciate what you have and go from there.*

I used to think if I did things for myself over others that I was being selfish. I wished someone told me that putting the focus on me was not a selfish act. How I did not see this is mind boggling. It's the airplane scenario. You need to put the oxygen mask on yourself before you put it on your child. If you do not take care of yourself, how will you be able to take care of others or be successful in what you do?

How about breathing? Who thinks about it? Usually, it is pretty automatic. If you start thinking about it, does it get harder to do? It is amazing how our breath can be used to improve focus and reduce stress.

Try out different breathing exercises like the box breath (my favorite!) and alternate nostril breathing to activate your parasympathetic nervous system, the "rest and digest" system. These exercises help reduce the effects of the sympathetic nervous system, which is what causes the "fight or flight" we feel in our bodies, causing stress and anxiety.

This practice will also help you become self-aware of how your body feels and lead to a sense of calm and relaxation.

Try some breathing exercises in a quiet place or private space.

> **Deep Breathing Exercise:** *Sit comfortably. Close your eyes, think of something pleasant, and begin to breathe in deeply through your nose, and exhale slowly through your mouth. Continue breathing in and out a few more times, focusing on how your breath makes you feel. Slowly go back to your natural breath and relax with your eyes closed for a minute or two before you slowly get back up.*

> **Box Breath Method:** *I use this breath often. Sit comfortably. Close your eyes, and think of something pleasant. Inhale deeply for a count of four, hold for a count of four, exhale for another count of four, and finally hold for a count of four. Repeat a couple of times. Slowly go back to your natural breath and relax with your eyes closed for a minute or two before you slowly get back up.*

> **Alternate Nostril Breathing:** *Sit comfortably. Put your thumb over your left nostril and inhale deeply through the right nostril. Hold for a few seconds, then release your thumb, close your right nostril, and exhale through your left nostril. Repeat several times, alternating nostrils. Slowly go back to your natural breath and relax with your eyes closed for a minute or two before you slowly get back up.*

Using some of these breathing techniques during physical exercise can help you feel better. Adding these breathing exercises to your yoga practice or simply focusing on your breath while running or being still in the moment can definitely give you a sense of calm.

Add these breathing exercises into your routines, and see how they will help you focus on YOU and bring calm to your day.

GROUNDING

Grounding, sometimes called earthing, is when you physically walk, stand, or do activities on the ground, sand, or in water and physically connect to the earth's natural energy. This connection is healthy for our bodies and can reduce stress.

I love doing things like gardening, and taking walks on a beach, but you can walk barefoot in the grass or swim in a natural lake to get the benefits of grounding.

Sometimes, when you are feeling stressed, or your body is in an anxious state, it can be difficult to calm yourself. There is a grounding technique you can do that may help. It is called the **54321 Method**. Here is how it works.

> *5 Find five things you can see: tree, door, etc.*
> *Say them out loud or to yourself.*
> *4 Find four things you can touch; chair, fence, etc.*
> *Touch them if possible.*
> *3 Find three things you can hear; bird, music, etc.*
> *2 Find two things you can smell; candle, food, etc.*
> *1 Find one thing you can taste; gum, fruit, etc.*

Doing these activities may help you and your body to calm down. Once my daughter was stuck on the L in Chicago underground and I went through this method with her to keep her calm. Keep it handy.

It is important to seek professional help if you are experiencing anxiety on a regular basis. Sometimes, it can be something you don't realize is causing it. Another tool you can use is the HALT system, an acronym for Hungry, Angry, Lonely, and Tired. Ask yourself these questions: Am I **Hungry**? Am I **Angry**? Am I **Lonely**? Am I **Tired**? If you are feeling any of these, what can you do immediately to help yourself?

Try to find the right system for you in bringing the focus on yourself. Improve your well-being by reducing stress, which is key to getting deeper in touch with yourself.

AL-ANON TWELVE-STEP PROGRAM

Let's talk a little about Al-Anon's 12 Steps. This program was designed for people living with loved ones having an unhealthy addiction and to learn how to cope with this. The steps provide techniques to help you through the frustration, anger, or the feeling of isolation. Rather than focusing on the person with the addiction and completely losing yourself, these steps are simply an excellent way to live your life day to day.

Finding your focus using Al-Anon's 12 Steps to put yourself first is a healthy addition to your toolbox.

Below is a brief introduction to each step:

> **Step 1:** *Admitting Powerlessness – This first step is powerful, an important understanding that you must come to terms with. You cannot control everything.*
> **Step 2:** *Belief in a Higher Power – The next step is putting your faith in a higher power. Letting go of control and having faith that all will work out.*
> **Step 3:** *Letting Go of Control – Do you see the theme here? Again, try to recognize that you cannot control other people.*
> **Step 4:** *Conducting a Moral Inventory – It is a time for you to truly, objectively dive deep into who you are.*
> **Step 5:** *Admitting Wrongdoing – The key is being completely honest with yourself, admit to any wrongdoing and open yourself up to forgiveness.*
> **Step 6:** *Ready for Change – This step keeps you moving forward; ready for new changes in your life.*
> **Step 7:** *Asking for Help – It allows you to be vulnerable and feel comfortable enough to begin asking for help.*
> **Step 8:** *Making Amends – Taking responsibility for your past actions. If it brings no harm, let them know how sorry you are and move on.*
> **Step 9:** *Continuing to Self-Reflect – Maintenance, continue growing, learning, and reflecting.*

Step 10: *Taking Responsibility –Find ways to keep yourself accountable and responsible for your actions.*
Step 11: *Seeking Spiritual Connection –Find ways to connect spiritually at a deeper level.*
Step 12: *Carrying the Message to Others –Show others that there are tools out there to help them and the people we love in our lives.*

To learn more about the Al-Anon program, go to https://al-anon.org/

JOYFUL PRACTICE

This exercise can be found in ***Chapter Eleven*** and will help you dig a little deeper into self-reflection using the Al-Anon 12 Steps.

All of us have beautiful similarities and differences. One common thread I've witnessed is the fact that we are putting others first. Our own needs are an afterthought.

How many times have you put your needs to the side? It isn't easy taking care of family, be it our parents, kids, or spouses. It is also stressful making sure you are the best you can be at work. Sometimes, it's trying to keep up with what you think everyone else is doing. You can lose yourself. I have done all of this in my lifetime.

It's important to take the time and energy to get to know what you need. Are you making yourself a priority, setting those boundaries, and finding the strength to say "no" when necessary without guilt? This is not easy to do. It's a "win" when you find the courage to say "no" to others. The uneasiness of how this may feel is well worth it in the long run.

The best thing about being focused on ourselves is that you start to know what you need. This can be the beginning of making better decisions, creating more meaningful relationships. You may find a new sense of purpose and direction that you didn't have before.

When that focus is brought to you, it will become stronger and bring a little spark of joy to your heart.

~

THINK ABOUT IT...

I want to be myself and be heard.

I want to find calm.

MY INTENTIONS...

I intend to focus on myself more.

CHAPTER 5

LETTING GO

SERENITY PRAYER

"God grant me the serenity To accept the things I cannot change,

Courage to change the things I can,

And the wisdom to know the difference.

Living one day at a time, Enjoying one moment at a time;

Accepting hardships as the pathway to peace."

— REINHOLD NIEBUHR (UNABRIDGED VERSION)

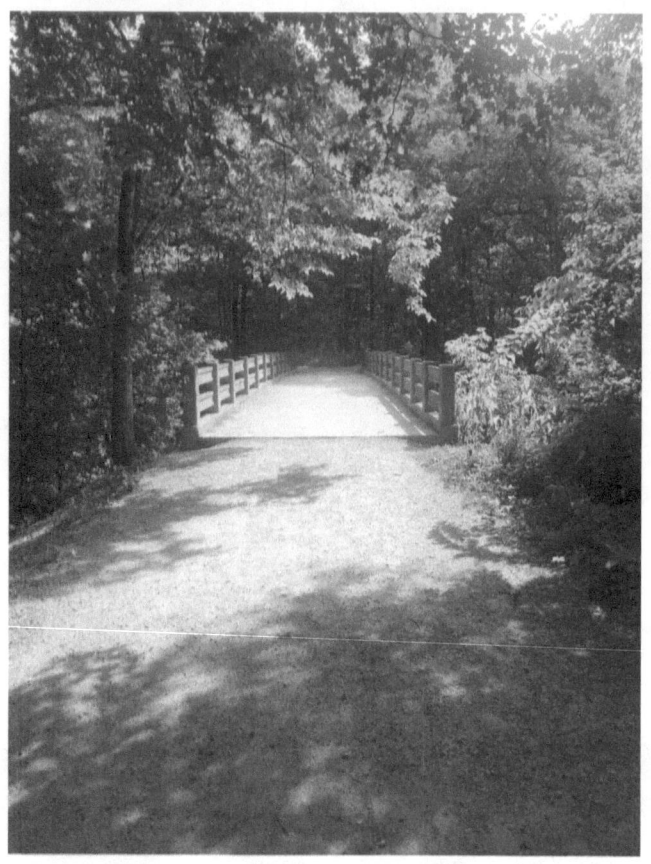

IT'S ALL RIGHT; GO AHEAD AND LET IT GO.

Think about how to let go of past relationships, false belief systems, or a poor self-image; We will dive in to understand how we can feel empowered and free when we begin to let go of these negative holds on us. What is holding you back from letting go? Clutter, Ugh! There are two kinds of clutter: physical and mental. Finally, we'll talk about the Alcoholics Anonymous (AA) 12-Step Program and how these steps can help anyone learn how to focus on themselves and thrive.

LET GO OF THE PAST

Letting Go of things can be difficult. Letting go of the past is a transformative experience. Your tightly held baggage may be holding you back. Are you stuck in repeat mode? Does something stop you every time you start to move forward? When you do not face your past, it can stop you from moving forward. Letting go provides the space for new adventures, well-deserved joy, and openness to new opportunities. Let go of the resentment, anger, and regret... It is incredibly freeing to let go of negatives that have a strong hold on our lives.

LET GO OF FEAR

Fear is real and will paralyze us. Allowing it to control means that everything you do is limited. It's as if you decide to check in with fear to see if it is ok before you go out and do something. It prevents you from reaching goals and to live out your dreams. *Get comfortable with the uncomfortable.* Oh, am I sick of hearing that one! This is the beginning of the self-growth you need to move on. Let go of the fear and feel the transformation taking place. Embracing the uncertainty, you will start to see life as an adventure full of well-deserved experiences and possibilities instead of doing the same thing over-and-over.

LET GO OF CONTROL

Try to relax. Take those deep, deep breaths and let go of that control you think you have. So many of us want to control everything in our lives, from our relationships, kids, and careers. Over-scheduling results in exhaustion. Do you think it is best to do it yourself and not involve others? I know I was a firm believer that it would take less time if I just did it myself and then I knew it was done right. If you feel the same way, I suggest re-evaluating.

How many times do you think you have control over a situation and watch it go in a completely different direction? This fantasy of control brings us the racing heartbeats and hyperventilation. Close your eyes, take a deep breath, and have faith that all will work out the way it should. *Letting Go* of that control! Our focus will return to what matters most to us and help change our mindset to positive behaviors and good decision-making processes.

Let Go of Perfectionism

I used to be proud that I was a perfectionist. It stopped me from feeling happy or excited or accomplishing something. I still struggle with this one at times. Embrace who you really are and begin to live into your authentic self. You will grow and start to enjoy what each day brings in a more mindful manner. *Letting Go* of perfection, allowing mistakes, and knowing you are human are the first steps. If you cannot do it perfectly, you feel best not to do it at all. So what if it isn't perfect! Just do it and let go of perfectionism.

Let Go of Expectations

Expectations can definitely be why you become disappointed and frustrated when something doesn't work out. *Letting Go* of your expectations and live in the moment. Have faith that it will work out and maybe even be better than you might have expected. Letting go of expectations will bring you a sense of calm and happiness instead of focusing on what can go wrong or getting triggered.

How many times have you not let yourself be excited about something because, in the back of your mind, you are afraid you might jinx something? **Let go**, breathe, and enjoy the moment.

Letting Go of the Physical Clutter

This *Letting Go* can be a transformative experience that can change how you look at things in life. Let go of your fear, the fake control, along with your expectations. Once you can do this, it will be amazing how you will begin to live a more fulfilling life with that **joy** you are searching for.

Letting go is a necessary step in the world of physical clutter. Many of us hold on to our stuff, whether it be clothes, books, or sentimental items, having painful or beautiful memories that we want to hold on to or can't **let go** of. When you do this, you lose opportunities to grow and have new experiences. It can be a good practice to try to work through these feelings and **let go** of the stuff you hold on to. I encourage my clients to focus on themselves as part of the organizing process. Can they identify their values, passions, and priorities? How does their physical space support the things they identify with? I help them create systems and routines that work for them rather than trying to fit into someone else's mold.

It's natural to feel some guilt in tossing away something someone gave you. You may feel an obligation to keep it. However, holding onto these items can weigh us down and prevent us from moving forward. I often hear from my clients, "My great aunt Mildred gave me that, and I can't get rid of it!" When your great aunt Mildred gave it to you, it might have been meaningful at the time. Memories are now in your mind and heart. They did not give it to you to be a burden, as you do not need to hold on to it forever if it is no longer used or you never even liked it. There are many other ways to preserve these memories.

Go through your stuff. Ask yourself what feelings come up when you see it or touch it. Let yourself feel those emotions. Ask yourself: does this object I am holding onto serve a sensible purpose? Sometimes, you can have a good feeling about giving something to someone else who really needs it and would be grateful to have it.

Feel the positive energy and the ability to think more clearly to enjoy what is most important to you in your life. Choose people and experiences over stuff.

As difficult as it is to let go of unnecessary stuff, doing so will help you confront the control you think you have. Letting go will allow us strength and begin to have the faith needed to know everything will be okay.

A huge part of the process is to be non-judgmental. Have supportive people to help you that will not make you feel insecure or bad about your decisions on whether to keep or toss something. Be kind to yourself; take baby steps.

Take a deep breath and see how you feel after letting something physical go. You will be surprised how good it feels.

BEYOND THE PHYSICAL CLUTTER

Knowing how physical clutter and our stuff can negatively affect our day-to-day life, there is another type of clutter that isn't always recognized. This is the mental clutter —racing thoughts, our ignored emotions or feelings, or digital clutter.

This mental clutter may be reliving an old experience from the past and trying to figure out why these things keep happening or what you could have done differently. These thoughts are triggered by something going on during the day without us even realizing it. Or we are having sleepless nights worrying about something we have no control over.

Having mental clutter can stop you from living the peaceful life you want to have. Physical clutter has negative effects in preventing us from growing, making good decisions, and living in the now; the same goes for mental clutter.

Holding onto unresolved thoughts or emotions will drain our bodies and minds. When we cannot come to terms with these feelings, we become bitter and stressed. Having negative thoughts prevents us from making healthy decisions and building good relationships.

Digital clutter as well can make you feel overwhelmed. How many emails do you have in your inbox? Are you able to get to them, or do you just ignore them? Do you participate in social media? All of these digital means will make you tired, heavy, and anxious, not to mention some are addictive.

Decluttering the physical and mental is a necessary process to sort through in order to begin living in the now and appreciating what you have. Using the tools discussed will help you create goals and strategies for living a decluttered life.

This might involve the practice of being mindful, using meditation to quiet the mind, seeking therapy or coaching to work through the emotional clutter. Whatever the approach, *the goal is to create more space.*

JOYFUL PRACTICE

Take a step back, identify the sources of clutter in your life, and take action for letting go.

Note what types of clutter you have currently in your life, physical or mental. List as many as you can think of. Next, determine an action that will help you remove this clutter. Finally, write down how you are feeling before and after each letting go.

Identify clutter in your life:	Action to let it go:	How I am feeling before and after:
Examples:		
I am constantly focused on a co-worker that is not nice to me.	*I will focus on my work tasks and not give my energy or attention to the co-worker.*	***Before**, I feel anxious about my co-worker's actions.* ***After** I begin to focus on me I felt good and relieved.*
_____	_____	_____
_____	_____	_____
_____	_____	_____
_____	_____	_____

Letting go is tough, regardless if it is physical or mental. The key take-away here is that you need to begin to develop strategies to help you move on to better decisions and habits to be able to move forward.

ALCOHOLICS ANONYMOUS TWELVE-STEP PROGRAM

We touched on the Al-Anon 12-Step Program. This similar program can be a powerful tool to help with addiction.

> **Step 1:** *Admitting Powerlessness –Let go of what you are powerless over. You must admit that you cannot control it. Through this process, you will begin to be open to change.*

Step 2: *Believing in a Higher Power –Believe there is a higher power.*

Step 3: *Turning Our Will Over to a Higher Power –Have faith through meditation and prayer or have a deeper connection with a higher power to help persevere.*

Step 4: *Taking a Moral Inventory –Think about our actions and behaviors. Patterns of our behavior may appear.*

Step 5: *Admitting Our Wrongs –Admitting our wrongs to ourselves, to a higher power, and to another person. This is hard!*

Step 6: *Being Willing to Let Go –Let go of our character defects. It's time to do the work in improving ourselves.*

Step 7: *Asking a Higher Power to Remove Our Shortcomings – Ask our higher power to remove these defects. Find humility; asking for help allows strength and courage to change.*

Step 8: *Making a List of Those We Have Harmed – Make a list of people you have harmed.*

Step 9: *Making Amends –Take responsibility for our actions and sincerely apologizing for what you have done.*

Step 10: *Continuing to Take Inventory –Continue to take inventory of yourself to avoid falling back into old patterns.*

Step 11: *Seeking Conscious Contact with a Higher Power –Take time each day to connect with your higher power and seek guidance and strength.*

Step 12: *Carrying the Message to Others –Share your experiences, strength, and hope with others and be a source of support and encouragement.*

To learn more about the 12 Steps of Alcoholics Anonymous (AA), go to: https://www.aa.org/the-twelve-steps

JOYFUL PRACTICE

This exercise can be found in **Chapter Eleven** and will give you more ways to **let go**.

Letting Go is a continuous process, and the steps of AA provide tools to help you keep on the path. By using these steps along with our other tools, you can continue to grow and let go. It takes time and effort, but with commitment and dedication to yourself, you can find peace and freedom in the process of letting go.

∽

THINK ABOUT IT...

I want to let go of the past in a healthy manner.

I want to let go of control.

I want to let go of expectations.

MY INTENTIONS...

I intend to begin to let go of my physical clutter.

CHAPTER 6

MAKING CHOICES

W hat are you willing to give up to have something else? When making decisions, consider the various aspects of your situation and have a good understanding of what you may need to give up.

It's time to do a deep dive into your values and priorities so that your choices clearly align with those values and beliefs. Two techniques for making good decisions are the *SWOT* Analysis and the Life Flow Chart Process.

SWOT ANALYSIS

A SWOT analysis is an acronym for **Strengths, Weaknesses, Opportunities, and Threats.** Use this tool when you need to explore what your situation is.

JOYFUL PRACTICE

Think about your situation or goal. Start to write down strengths you may find in this situation. Next, write down all the weaknesses you can think of. Then, write down the opportunities you find and any threats. You can write down multiple answers.

Below is an example:

Use the four squares to write in all Strengths, Weaknesses, Opportunities, and Threats associated with the decision you are working on. In our example, only one is written for each category. You can write down multiple answers.

You are thinking about taking out a home equity loan to remodel your home.

STRENGTHS	WEAKNESSES
We will build more equity in our home once the remodeling is complete.	We will have a higher mortgage payment and may need to give up extra activities such as travel.
OPPORTUNITIES	THREATS
We will now have enough space to enjoy more activities in our home together as a family.	If one of us lost our job, it may be difficult to keep up with the mortgage.

Once you have completed your SWOT Analysis, you can move on to your Pros and Cons list. Think about how your decisions impact you and everyone else involved. Trust your instincts or gut feelings, along with the facts.

PRO'S & CON'S

>   **Pro-Strengths:** We are Increasing our Equity.
>   **Con-Strengths:** Living in the house during construction is not ideal.

Pro-Weaknesses: We can be mindful of how we spend money.
Con-Weaknesses: We may disagree on how we spend money.

Pro-Opportunities: More Family Time/Entertaining.
Con-Opportunities: The cost to entertain may be high.

Pro-Threats: Find a higher-paying job.
Con-Threats: Work multiple jobs to pay bills or ask for help.

Don't let fear drive your decisions. Changing your mind, saying no, or revising the plan is okay. Remember to be sure your decision still aligns with your goals and values. If it doesn't feel right, it probably isn't. Consider the short - and long-term - consequences of all your choices in your decision-making process. Circumstances may change and, therefore, your decisions may as well. It's okay to take risks and make mistakes as long as you are learning from them. Embrace the opportunities that come when making your decisions.

LIFE FLOW CHART PROCESS - OVERVIEW

What is the Life Flow Chart Process? Something I invented to help my clients. This all-inclusive tool will help you in creating goals that align with your values and beliefs. Along with other practices to keep you on track, this is a fantastic maintenance tool as well. Let's look at the following list of steps that will help you continue to have the focus on YOU.

1. Know your top five goals. (Are these PACT Goals)? [Revisit Chapter 3]
2. Identify what your values and beliefs are.
3. Practice self-reflection. Be mindful of the consequences of your decision-making.
4. Practice self-care activities.
5. Let go of negative thoughts and emotions in a healthy manner.
6. Practice gratitude.
7. Surround yourself with a network of supportive people.

8. Protect your mental health.
9. Seek continuous improvement.
10. Celebrate your wins.

The Life Flow Chart Process assists us in making the right choices, moving us along our Joy Journey.

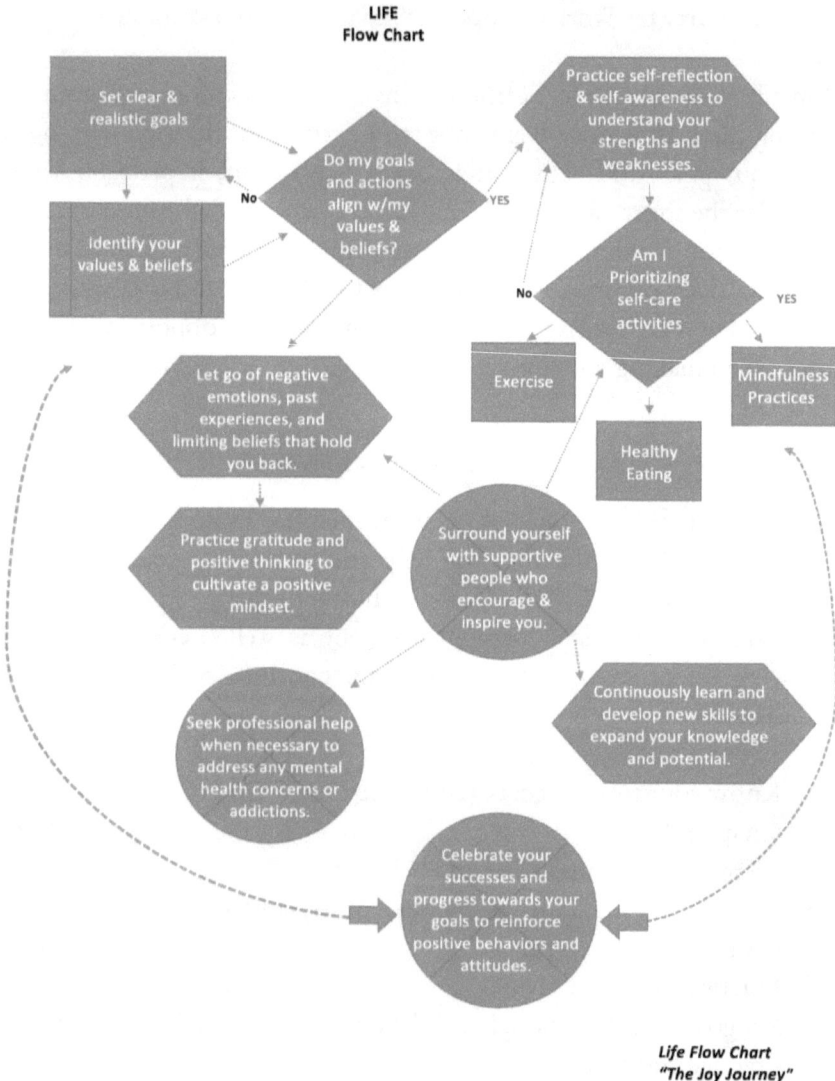

Life Flow Chart
"The Joy Journey"

Bear in mind this is an extremely personal process. Self-reflection, soul-searching, and a clear understanding of what matters to you helps. This next exercise gives you the opportunity to dive deep into your values and beliefs by answering questions in detail.

JOYFUL PRACTICE

This exercise can be found in **Chapter Eleven** and will help you get into more details in various areas in your daily life.

THIS IS IT! Utilizing the LIFE Flow Chart Process in more detail will give you the ultimate tool from your toolbox to live the life you deserve. When you feel like something isn't right or you are losing what you have obtained thus far, make adjustments. Go through the LIFE Flow and see what you are missing.

The Life Flow Chart kit available soon (www.lettuceorganize.com) to post on your wall to keep track of your progress and maintain what you have created.

～

Think About It...

I want to know what I am giving up.

I want to have confidence in my decision-making.

I want to understand my choices.

My Intentions...

I intend to practice more self-care.

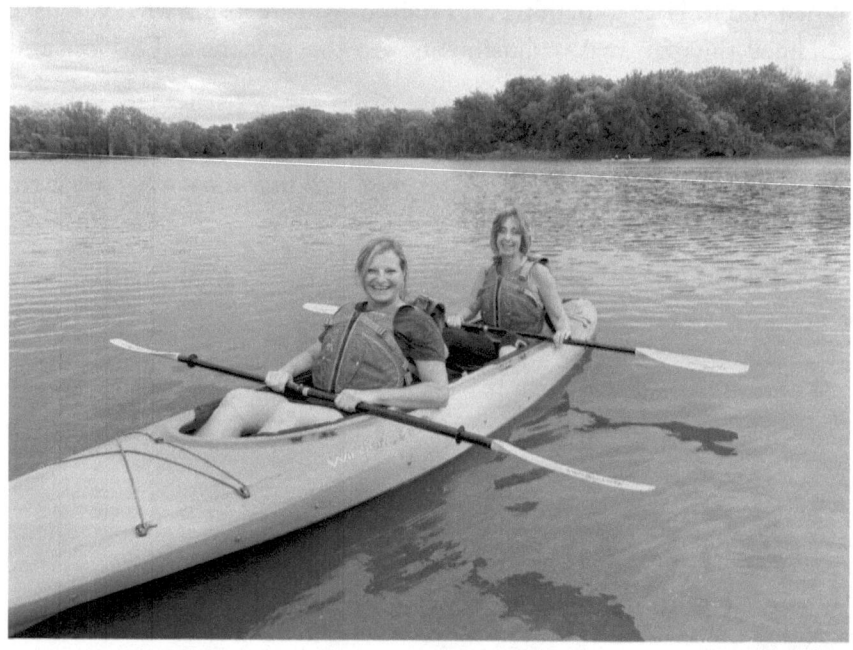

CHAPTER 7

SET ME FREE

Having accountability can be hard if you do not have someone holding a deadline in your face. We will use an Accountability Chart to help us be accountable to ourselves. We will also look at a few healing practices that will be a great addition to our routine. These practices will allow you to naturally release the stress and tension running through your body, giving you the freedom to relax and just breathe.

ACCOUNTABILITY CHART

An Accountability Chart is a valuable tool for examining daily habits and determining what you are actually spending time on.

Try to fill out an Accountability Chart for two weeks. This timeframe should be good enough to gather most of the information on what you are doing. Completing the chart will allow you to analyze what tasks you are doing. In doing this you will see if they are valuable and necessary. See if these tasks can be given to someone else, giving you more time and freedom to do other things.

This exercise can be found in **Chapter Eleven** and will not only help you determine how you are spending your time, but it will also help you evaluate what changes are needed.

Look for patterns. See who is doing what. Look at your daily activities and see if someone else can take on that responsibility. Doing the exercise for at least two weeks, you can cover most, if not all, of what you do. Using this tool will also help you look into your current tasks and rethink whether they are necessary or bring value to your day-to-day life.

Remember, setting yourself free is a process that takes time and effort but, with determination, we can achieve our goals, live the life we desire, and have that spark of joy in our journey!

Next page is a sample Accountability Chart.

Name — Date - Frequency / Weekly Daily Hourly / M T W Th F Sat Sun	When? Day / Time	Add details to what you are doing?	Getting Ready for work	Making breakfast	Making Lunches	Dropping kids off to school	Driving to w...
Who is doing it?	When? Day / Time	Add details to what you are doing?					
Me	Monday 5:00 am	Taking shower/ finding clothes / getting my workstuff together					
Me	Monday 6:30 am			Making me, my partner and kids breakfast			
Me	Monday 7:00 am				Making Lunches for me, my partner and kids		
Me	Monday 7:30 am					Dropping kids to their schools or daycare	

TAPPING

Tapping (Emotional Freedom Techniques (EFT)) is a practice that focuses on pressure points on the body to alleviate hidden trauma and unrelieved stress and help relax the tension flowing through your body.

Tapping is a powerful subconscious reprogramming tool. A combination of energy work (utilizing acupressure points), psychology, and affirmations. This mind-body method rapidly reduces stress and trauma while increasing calm in the body and mind.

If you've ever found yourself losing sleep due to worry, replaying a breakup in your mind or a hurtful comment that someone said to you, you're in luck. All of these situations (plus countless more) can be radically improved and transformed with Tapping.

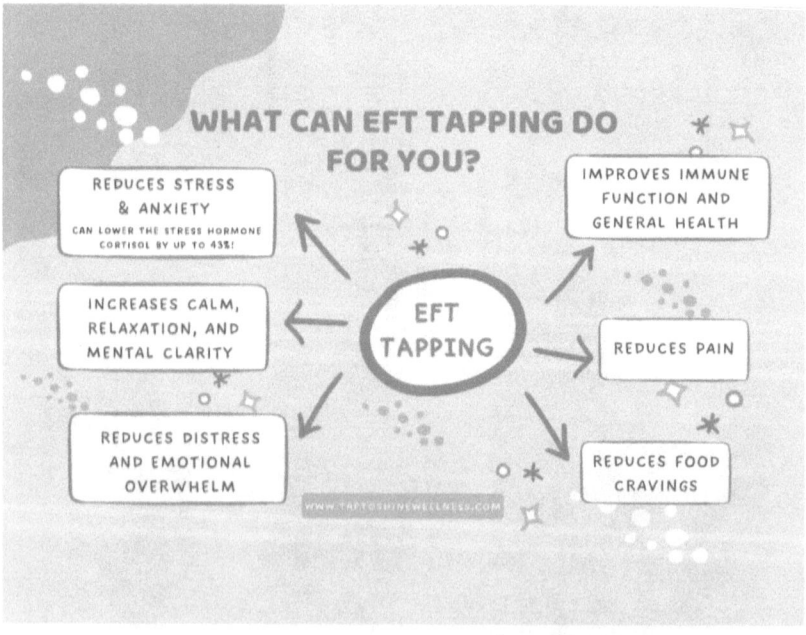

Photo Credit: Sonya Pietruszka

The name Emotional Freedom Techniques is no misnomer. Freedom is truly what you get. When implemented correctly, the result is freedom from the issue that is causing you distress. Moreover, you will feel lighter, more relaxed, and more peaceful in your body and mind.

What does a tapping practice look like? As the name suggests, you physically tap with your fingertips on different acupressure points on your face and upper torso, while voicing statements out loud.

The first step in the process is to identify your issue of concern. This can literally be anything. Maybe you feel angry or annoyed with your partner/spouse/kid/friend/etc. Or you can't get the memory of a bad experience out of your mind and it's causing you to feel anxious. Or perhaps you're feeling resistance around cleaning out your closet, and it's keeping you stuck. Whatever it is, if there's an emotion around it, you can tap on it.

Once you identify the issue you want to focus on, the next step is to identify the emotion(s) that come up for you when you think about the issue. There may be more than one emotion that surfaces, and that's okay. Note them all down.

Next, determine where you feel each emotion in your body. You might notice a heaviness in your gut, like a "rock in your stomach" or a pressure or tightness in the chest. You may or may not notice a physical sensation in the body at all, and that's okay! Sometimes, we don't realize we're holding tension in the body until it releases during tapping. This is all part of the practice of connecting with the body.

The last pre-tapping step is to measure how big the emotion (and/or physical sensation) feels on a scale of 0–10, with 10 being high. You can think of it as **0 = "whatever, it doesn't bother"** and **10 = "worst thing ever."** In the case of more than one emotion, you will need to measure and get a number for each. The highest number is generally what you will start with.

Please note: *It is recommended that any issues you choose to work on are lower in numerical value (6 or below). Working with a certified EFT tapping practitioner on higher ranking issues (7+) is strongly recom-*

mended, especially for those new to Tapping, as more advanced techniques may be required.

Now for the tapping!

Each round of tapping starts on the side of the hand (SOH, see diagram), as you voice a set up statement out loud, three times. The formula for a basic set up statement is: "Even though" + problem or issue + affirmation. All you have to do is insert the emotion or physical sensation that is showing up for you.

Even though I feel <u><negative emotion></u> I fully love and accept myself.

After you finish saying the setup statement while tapping on the side of the hand, you will move to the top of the head and work your way down the body. Using your first and second fingers to tap on the acupressure points, you will say a word or short phrase at each tapping point to help keep your attention on the issue.

The tapping points and their abbreviations are as follows:

Top of head / Crown - **TOH**
Eyebrow - Start of your eyebrow, where the nose meets the brow - **EB**
Side of the Eye - Next to the outside corner of the eye, on the orbital bone - **SE**
Under the Eye - On the orbital bone, in line with pupil - **UE**
Under the Nose - Directly between nose and top lip - **UN**
Chin - Under the mouth, chin crease - **CH**
Collarbones - Down and out ~1 inch from the knobby start of the collarbones - **CB**
Under the Arm - Roughly 4 inches below the armpit, on the midseam of the body - **UA**
Side of the Hand - Fleshy part of the hand between the wrist and pinky joint - **SOH**

Once you finish a round of tapping, take a deep breath in through your nose, exhale through your mouth like you're blowing out a candle, and notice how you feel. You may need to do a couple more rounds of tapping depending on how much your number (0-10 measurement) has changed. The main goal is to reduce the emotional charge around the issue. Take your time with it, and give yourself permission to come back to it later, or seek help from a professional if you're not getting results by yourself.

JOYFUL PRACTICE

This exercise can be found in **Chapter Eleven** and will allow you to get the feel of Tapping.

How did it go? If you want to learn more about EFT, feel free to go to the links below.

Sonia Pietruszka, Certified EFT Tapping
Practitioner & Energy Makeover Coach
www.taptoshinewellness.com
IG: @TaptoShineWellness
FB: Tap to Shine Wellness
Youtube: @TaptoShineWellness

SOUND BATH MEDITATION

By Marilyn Metz, Founder of Star Sound Baths LLC
www.StarSoundBaths.com

Meditation is a transformative mindfulness practice that helps relieve stress, sharpen focus, and ground you in the present moment. In our fast-paced world, it offers a rare moment to pause and intentionally check in with yourself—something often overlooked amid the daily hustle. With so many responsibilities on your shoulders—balancing work, family, friends, and countless other roles—it's easy to feel overwhelmed. When stress piles up, it can spill over in unexpected ways: strained relationships, emotional overload, and even a weakened immune system.

Meditation invites you to slow down, release the demands of the outside world, and focus on you. It's a practice of self-awareness, guiding you to check in with your mental, emotional, and physical states. This awareness helps you take control of your well-being, shifting you from a reactive mindset to one of conscious response. While meditation is often associated with "quieting the mind," it's really about tuning into what your mind and body are telling you. This simple practice is known for its scientifically supported ability to calm the body's stress response, leaving you feeling more calm and present.

Sound Bath—also known as Sound Healing or Sound Meditation—is a unique form of meditation that incorporates the power of sound. In a sound bath, participants settle into a comfortable position, relaxing as they are immersed in the invisible force of sound vibrations from instruments like Crystal Singing Bowls, Tibetan Bowls, and Gongs. These immersive experiences are offered in both live and virtual settings, providing an accessible meditation method, especially for beginners. Sound gives the mind a gentle focal point, while the vibrations guide the body into deeper states of relaxation, amplifying the stress-relieving effects of meditation.

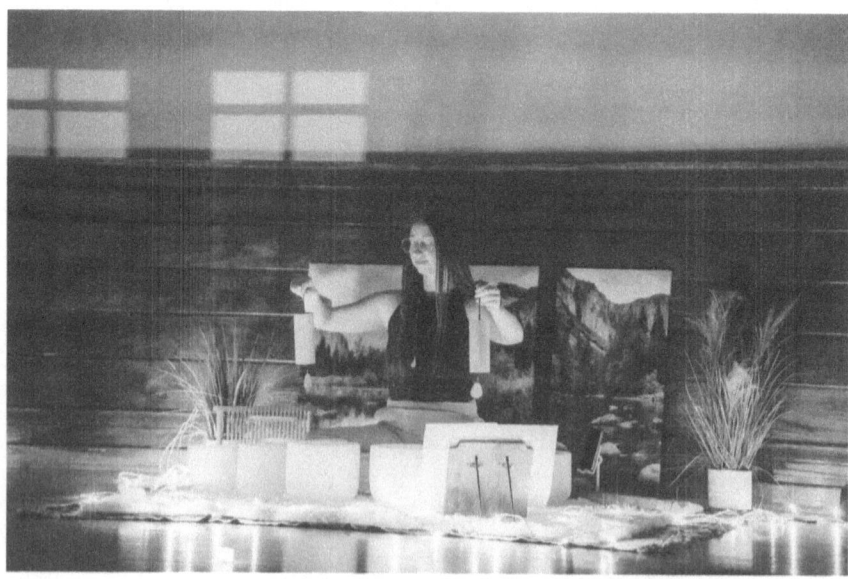

I utilize all of these practices to **Set Me Free**! You can too!

THINK ABOUT IT...

I want to know how I am spending my time.

I want to know who should be helping me.

I want to know if my activities are worthwhile.

MY INTENTIONS...

I intend to try some of these new relaxation techniques.

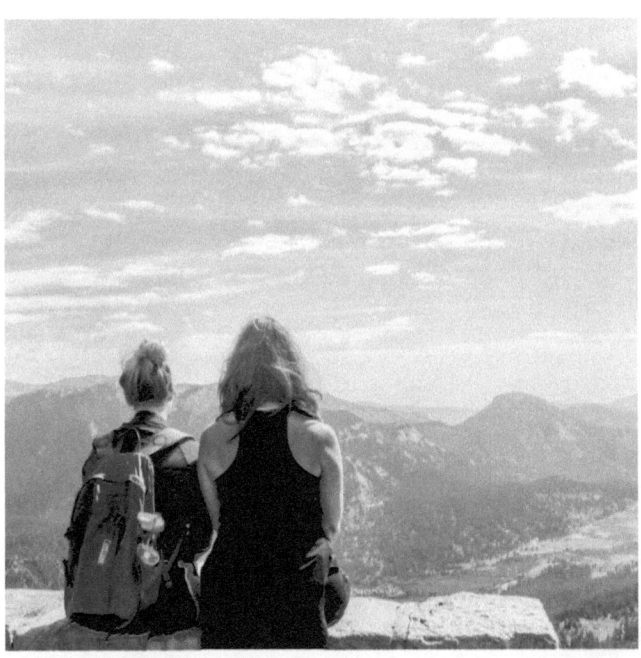

CHAPTER 8

THIS IS IT

SPARK OF JOY

W here to sit? Despite knowing I am having that little tickle in my chest, I will not acknowledge it and continue breathing deeply before boarding.

It's time, and we make our way to the back of the small plane. I sit, place my overstuffed backpack under the seat in front of me. I scramble to find my headphones; Open my CALM app to listen to the *Coastline at Sunset* in the background of everything else. "Flight Attendants, take your seats as we are ready for take-off." I breathe again once I hear the carts of the flight attendants bringing beverages throughout the aisle.

The plane begins to sway and bump, and I snuggle my head deep into the nook of my husband's shoulder, thoughts racing in my head. I begin to think of what I am grateful for. Interestingly enough, my gratitude list has grown as I get older. I begin to relax.

The pilot instructs the flight attendants to prepare for landing and, soon after, I feel the landing gear pop. I glance out the window, see we are there. As we slightly sway from side to side, we feel the wheels hit the pavement to a quick stop. I look at my husband, thank him for the trip he planned for us.

We make our way to the baggage claim area. I have a little skip to my step. We pass a typical O'Hare- Airport-stern-faced security guard, our eyes briefly meeting. He gives me a wink; it warms my soul. He sees the tiny spark of joy I found on this flight.

The key takeaway from this story: before you close your eyes tonight, write one thing you are grateful for, and sleep on it. You will find this is all you need to get that extra Spark of Joy and add a little skip to your step.

Someone asked me once: how do you know what Joy feels like? To really feel Joy, do you need to have the experience of feeling sorrow?

My Grateful List

Sorrow and joy's relationship can be, at best, convoluted as it will vary from person to person. Experiencing sorrow or sadness can bring more appreciation to feel a deeper joy. The distinction between sorrow and joy can make joy feel more intense and have a deeper meaning.

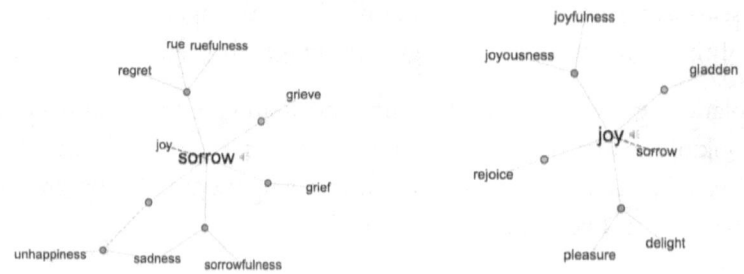

Visual Thesaurus. (n.d.). Synonym for "sorrow", "joy"

It is not written in stone that you must feel sorrow to experience joy. It depends on our emotional threshold and the coping mechanisms we've created through our experiences. We might find joy in the simplest things and have little experience with deep sorrow. In contrast, others might need to navigate through these knotty emotions to appreciate moments of happiness.

It can depend on the complexity of the emotions and what can influence them. The influencer list can be long depending on our own individual personality, our life experiences, and cultural background, etc. You might find that your capacity for joy is enhanced after overcoming sorrow, while other times you might find joy in everyday moments without necessarily experiencing profound sadness.

In essence, the relationship between sorrow and joy is highly individual, and can't be simplified into a rigidly strict rule. We all have diverse emotional experiences; what brings joy to one person may not be the same for another.

How can *you* find joy in your journey?

Joy is not constant and will come and go. Use the tools to be comfortable with who you are, and create the life you desire. **You deserve this!** Observing the little things in life can bring a spark of joy through your daily routines and eventually will last a lifetime.

Hold on to every spark of joy, live in the moment, feel and process what is happening around you. Use the tools that work to bring you joy in your journey. This is it!

~

THINK ABOUT IT...

I want to maintain what I created.

I want to live according to my Values and Beliefs.

I am finding Joy in my journey.

MY INTENTIONS...

I intend to hold on to happy moments.

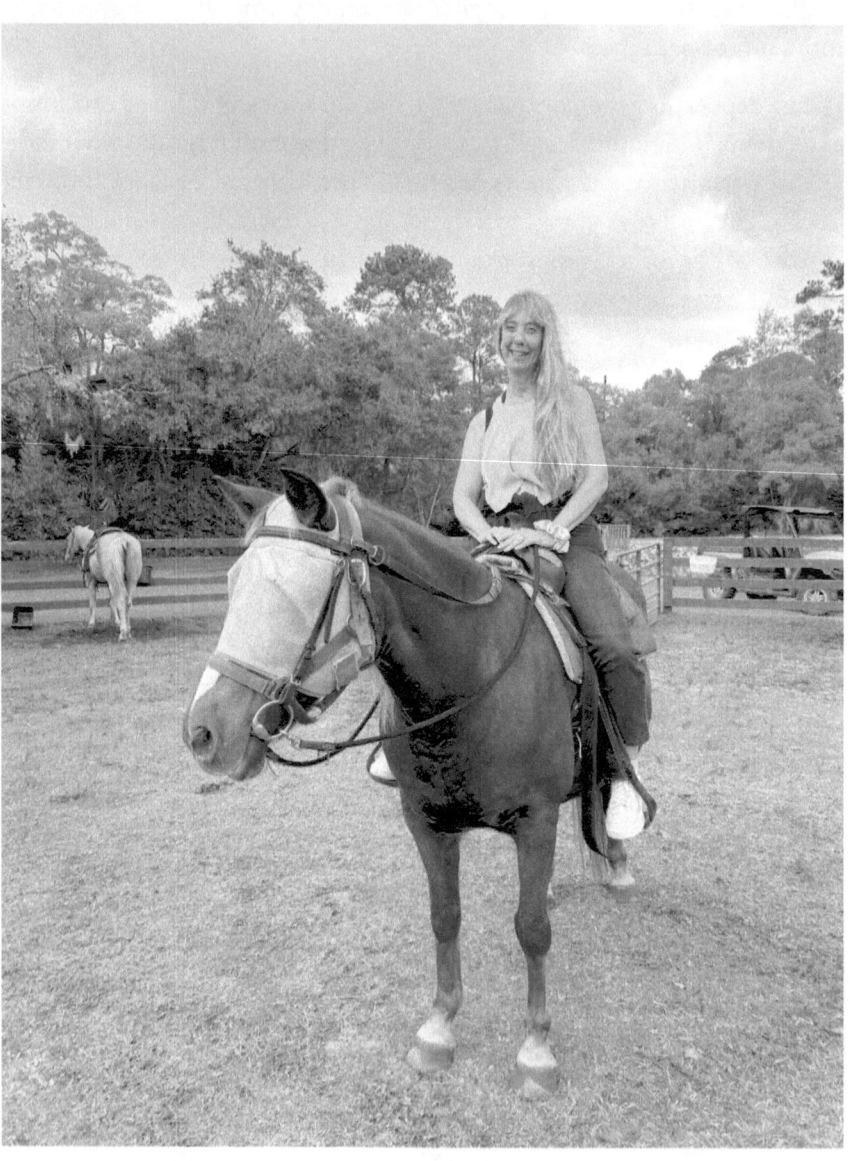

CHAPTER 9

YOU GOT THIS

YOU'VE GOT THIS

"You are more~
More than you believed yourself to be
You would see the beauty of who you are
If you could see what it is we see.

We're here to let you know
That we believe in you
You've got this, you can do it
Let your resilience shine through.
We're the people in your corner
Who support and cheer you on.
You go girl, you've got this
Be who you are, be strong."

— GAYLE MCMILLAN

TOOLBOX WHEEL

Find the System that Works **Best** for You!

READJUSTMENT STEPS	A COSIER LIFE	The LIFE FLOW CHART
Review	Activity	Top Five Goals
Values & Beliefs	Conveyance	Determine
Identify	Obstruction	Self-Reflection
Resolve	Shortcoming	Self-Care
Redesign	Irrelevant	Let Go of Negativity
Prioritize	Excess	Practice Gratitude
Maintenance	Reserve	Resources
		Mental Health

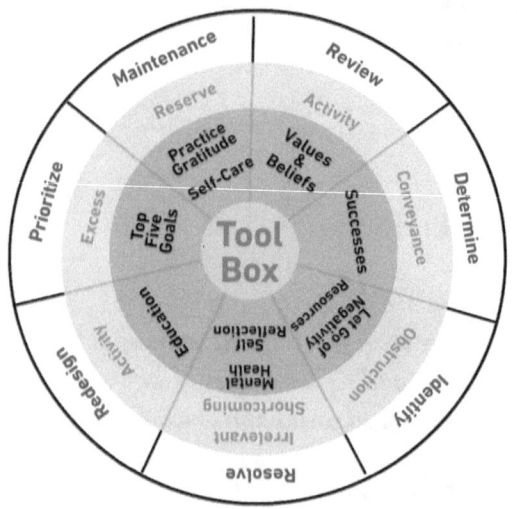

I combined the framework you have learned in the previous chapters, such as the **Seven Readjustment Steps**: *Review, Determine, Identify, Resolve, Redesign, Prioritize, and Maintenance* (which may be used to help structure your effectiveness in improving your daily life), with **A COSIER Life** (which is our seven wastes): *activity, conveyance, obstruction, shortcoming, irrelevant, excess, and reserve* and finally the **Life Flow Chart Process** to create the *Tool Box Wheel*, which will help you focus on the steps that may need extra attention. You can spin the wheel and choose three from each system you might want to work on.

Utilizing the **Tool Box Wheel** will allow you to combine the specific tools you want to focus on easily to fine tune your *Liveable Plan*.

Utilize all or some of the tools in the Toolbox to reach your goals. Following the Illustration of the Wheel, we can combine ***one slice at a time***. Recognize the connection between these categories. We can choose any of the tools from the three categories.

Below shows how to utilize all three systems together to help us make time for ourselves. This is the first piece of the pie. In this scenario, the following has been chosen from **The Life Flow** (Practice Gratitude & Self Care), from **The Seven Wastes** (Reserve) and from the **Seven Readjustment Steps** (Maintenance). Through these choices, we are able to focus entirely on how we can work at making time for ourselves. Practice and reinforcement of these specific tools make it happen!

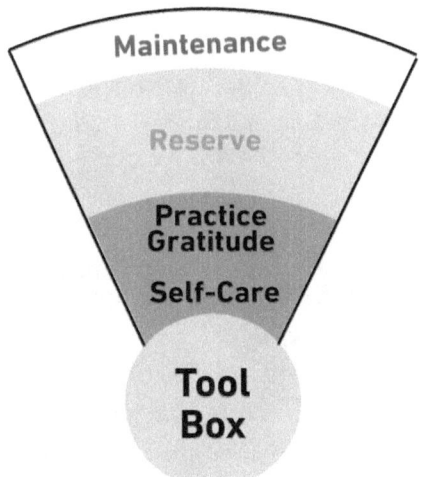

MAINTENANCE

> ***Consistency:*** *To sustain improvements in your life periodically revisit your goals. Track your progress, and make necessary adjustments.*
> ***Self-Care:*** *Have self-care practices scheduled in your daily routine to give you the energy and resilience to pursue your goals.*

Example Answer: *I will continue to schedule 20 minutes a day on my phone calendar first thing in the morning to take a walk and do deep breathing.*

RESERVE

> **Emergency Financial Fund:** *Build an emergency fund in times of unexpected expenses.*
> **Energy Management:** *Avoid overcommitting yourself, and take breaks to recharge when needed.*
> **Time Buffer:** *Leave some time in your schedule to accommodate the unexpected. This prevents over-scheduling and reduces stress. Work towards personal improvement to have a more fulfilling and balanced life. Improvement is an ongoing process; adapting these principles to our specific needs is key to success.*

Example Answer: *I will say* **"no"** *when I am exhausted and use the extra time I might have to do something for myself.*

PRACTICE GRATITUDE

> **Gratitude Journal:** *Keep a gratitude journal. Regularly write down things you are thankful for.*
> **Express Gratitude:** *Express your gratitude to others. A simple "thank you" makes a difference in how you and others feel.*
> **Gratitude Rituals:** *Incorporate gratitude into your daily routine, such as expressing how thankful you are before meals or bedtime.*

SELF CARE

> **Physical Health:** *Exercise regularly, eat nutritious meals, and get enough sleep. Physical well-being impacts your overall life satisfaction.*

Relaxation: Incorporate relaxation techniques such as yoga, meditation, or hobbies into your routine.
Set Boundaries: Learn to say "no" when necessary. Setting boundaries protects your time and energy.

Example Answer: *I will begin to journal again. I haven't been doing it; I know this will help my mood.*

These connections should reflect our goals, beliefs, and passions. They will evolve as we move through life's journey. Stay focused and positive, open to change when needed. The Toolbox Wheel is here as a guide to bring you to action that will improve your daily life.

JOYFUL PRACTICE

This exercise can be found in **Chapter Eleven** and should guide you to improve your daily life.

How did it go? Have you noticed that throughout this book, you are on a repeat cycle? We should begin to see a new pattern of behavior of who we want to be and bring a **spark of joy** into our everyday routines.

If not, reevaluate your behaviors and goals using the framework in these exercises so you can begin to systematically assess, plan, and implement improvements in the areas needed.

Remember that personal growth is an ongoing process that can help you stay focused and organized on your journey to a better life. By staying adaptable, and positive, you guide your actions and ultimately improve your life. **You Got This**!

The ToolBox Wheel kit available soon (www.lettuceorganize.com*).*

THINK ABOUT IT...

I want it to feel natural to use these various tools.

I want to use what I need to improve myself.

I will use the system that works for me.

MY INTENTIONS...

I intend to use the tools that work best for me.

CHAPTER 10

KEEP IT GOING

Let's use simple templates that will help you do check-ins on how you're doing daily, weekly, monthly, quarterly, and yearly. To keep what you created going is the purpose of the following templates. Finally! You're now able to stay on track with your new lifestyle changes. This maintenance will involve consistent effort and commitment.

Reflect: Think about what is working well and what challenges you may be facing. Be aware of when or how to make adjustments to the plan to stay on track.

Goals: Take the time to regularly review goals and assess your progress. Make any adjustments to reflect changing priorities and circumstances. Look to these changes as an opportunity.

Habits: Consistently work to establish these new life-changing behaviors to become new, simple habits. Consistency is key to incorporating new habits into the daily or weekly routine. The more integrated they become, the easier they will be to maintain.

Accountability: When we have accountability, we feel encouraged, and motivation will surely increase.

Sharing what you're doing with a friend or close family member that you trust can be one way to stay accountable. Utilize apps to track your progress.

Celebrate your wins: Celebrate your successes and progress towards your goals to reinforce positive behaviors and attitudes. Acknowledge and celebrate small victories along the way. You are worth it! No matter what the milestone, it is important to feel the victory. Recognizing your progress will motivate you, and reinforce your commitment to your desired lifestyle.

Maintenance is an ongoing process. It's okay to get interrupted when you encounter new or unexpected challenges. When this happens, embrace it, be kind to yourself, and stay adaptable. You can **Keep It Going**!

JOYFUL PRACTICE

Here are some example checklists that will assist you in your maintenance program. In the blank spaces, create your own maintenance checklist. Do this for all the Maintenance Checklists.

DAILY MAINTENANCE

Sleep	7-9 hours of sleep a night		Is my sleep schedule consistent?	Yes No
Physical Activity	30 minutes of moderate exercise		Am I walking or taking the stairs when I can? Am I incorporating simple movement into my daily schedule?	Yes No Yes No
Healthy Eating	Incorporating healthy eating habits		Am I getting fruits, vegetables, whole grains, lean proteins, and healthy fats	Yes No

What other daily activities do you need to add here that will keep you on track?

WEEKLY MAINTENANCE

Social Connections	Schedule time with friends and family.		Am I spending quality time with friends and family?	Yes No
			Am I connecting with loved ones through calls, video chats, or in-person interactions?	Yes No
Hobbies & Leisure	Engage in activities you enjoy for relaxation and enjoyment.		Am I taking time to enjoy doing my hobbies?	Yes No
			Am I fostering a sense of enjoyment through these activities?	Yes No
Screen Time	Incorporate Limitations on screen time.		Am I on my social media too much?	Yes No
			Have I incorporated any tech-free breaks?	Yes No

What other weekly activities do you need to add here that will keep you on track?

MONTHLY MAINTENANCE

Goal Review	Review short-term and long-term goals set.		Do I have goals set?	Yes No
			Am I adjusting any of my goals when necessary?	Yes No
Self-Reflection	Reflect on your emotional well-being and overall satisfaction with life.		Do I have any areas in my life that I want to improve?	Yes No
			Do I have any strategies set to improve my personal growth?	Yes No

What other monthly activities do you need to add here that will keep you on track?

QUARTERLY MAINTENANCE

Health Check-ups	Schedule regular health check-ups and screenings.	Am I taking care of myself? Am I addressing any current health issues?	Yes No Yes No
Stress Assessment	Regularly evaluate the sources of the stress in your life.	Do I have any stress management techniques? Am I aware of the stresses in my life?	Yes No Yes No

What other quarterly activities do you need to add here that will keep you on track?

YEARLY MAINTENANCE

Professional Support	Schedule regular mental health check-ups once a year if needed.	Do I have a professional I can talk with about my mental health? Am I addressing my current mental health issues?	Yes No Yes No
Gratitude Practice	Regularly practice gratitude.	Do I have to reflect on the positive aspects of my life? Do I consistently journal?	Yes No Yes No
Review and Update Lifestyle Choices	Assess lifestyle choices.	Do I need to make any lifestyle adjustments to be sure I am accommodating my needs and goals set?	Yes No

What other yearly activities do you need to add here that will keep you on track?

Creating meaningful checklists can be a valuable tool. Try tailoring these to your Life Chart, to incorporate your top five achievable goals.

THINK ABOUT IT...

I want to be on top of my goals.

I want to be consistent on my check-ins.

I want to maintain what I created.

MY INTENTIONS...

I intend to maintain what I created.

CHAPTER 11

JOYFUL PRACTICES

I AM

> *"I know not whence I came,*
>
> *I know not whither I go;*
>
> *But the fact stands clear that I am here*
>
> *In this world of pleasure and woe.*
>
> *And out of the mist and murk*
>
> *Another truth shines plain –*
>
> *It is in my power each day and hour*
>
> *To add to its joy or its pain."*

— ELLA WHEELER WILCOX

Joyful Practice exercises live here. Try them as you go through each chapter. ***Take what works for you.*** Come back and revisit the others later if you want to give it another try.

Chapter Two - The Seven Readjustment Steps

This Joyful Practice will explore each Readjustment Step more deeply. Write your answers or thoughts for each step on a separate piece of paper. Use the grids on the following pages for your final answers.

~

Using the area below, start with *Step One, Review.*

Step One - Review

Review various areas of your life. (Create categories: Home, Work, Family, Wellness, Etc.) Think about what you are proud of. Think about your challenges.

On a separate piece of paper or use the space below to write out your answers or thoughts for Step One.

Category Examples:
    Kids, Mental Health, Diet, Partner, Religion, Job, Company,
    Myself, Family, Friends, Exercise, Networking, Money, Parents

BRAIN DUMP

∾

**Using the grid below, begin to write down
your answers for *Step Two - Determine*.**

The Seven Readjustment Steps
Step Two - Determine

Determine which aspects of your life are most relevant and your
biggest priorities. Review your list in Step One; identify and narrow
your list to what is most significant to your daily life.

On a separate piece of paper or use the space below to write
out your answers or thoughts for Step Two.

Examples:

My Kids
Step 2

Myself
Step 2

Enter your answer to *Step Three,*
***Identify Problems* into the grid below.**

The Seven Readjustment Steps

Step Three - Identify Problems

What issues/challenges continuously show up? For example:
Maybe you always run out of time for yourself, empty of energy
or passion to put toward your priorities.

On a separate piece of paper or use the space below to write
out your answers or thoughts for Step Three.

Examples:

My Kids	Too Many Activities
Step 2	**Step 3**

Myself	No Self Care / No Time for Me
Step 2	**Step 3**

Enter your resolutions in *Step Four, Resolve* into the grid below.

The Seven Readjustment Steps

Step Four - Resolve the Problem

What options do you have? What possible solutions could help?
What is in your control? What support systems are you working with?

On a separate piece of paper or use the space below to write
out your answers or thoughts for Step Four.

Examples:

My Kids	Too Many Activities	Re-evaluate Current Activities
Step 2	Step 3	Step 4

Myself	No Self Care / No Time for Me	Commit to having a specified amount of time for only me.
Step 2	Step 3	Step 4

Add the answer to *Step Five, your Redesign* column in the grid below, which will become your new habit.

The Seven Readjustment Steps

Step Five - Redesign Processes in Your Life

This will become your new habit. Visualize what your life might look like if you did things differently. Is there anywhere you can simplify? What small changes might have a big impact? For example, if you need more time to yourself, consider getting up 30 minutes earlier to enjoy your favorite morning drink in your favorite cozy spot at home. Doing just one simple task for yourself each day can make a difference.

On a separate piece of paper or use the space below to write out your answers or thoughts for Step Five.

Examples:

My Kids	Too Many Activities	Re-evaluate Current Activities	Add more quality time with kids, go to parks or museums, and work on home projects together
Step 2	Step 3	Step 4	Step 5

Myself	No Self Care / No Time for Me	Commit to having a specified amount of time for only me.
Step 2	Step 3	Step 4

Get up 1 hour earlier each morning and meditate.
Step 5

Once you have completed Steps One through Five, *Prioritize them in Step Six*. Finally *Step Seven - Maintenance*, write down ways you can support yourself in being successful to maintain your efforts.

The Seven Readjustment Steps

Step Six - Prioritize
Think about what's most important to you. Choose one thing to work towards at a time so you don't overwhelm yourself.

On the previous page (Step 5), Prioritize which redesign you want to work on first.

Examples:

Myself	No Self Care / No Time for Me	Commit to having a specified amount for me.
Step 2	**Step 3**	**Step 4**

Get up 1 hour earlier each morning and meditate.
Step 5

My Maintenance Plan Step 7: I am dealing with time constraints. I am serious about making "me" a priority. I will set an alarm on my phone and put it on my calendar.

My Kids	Too Many Activities	Re-evaluate Current Activities	Add more quality time with
Step 2	**Step 3**	**Step 4**	the kids. Go to the parks or museums and work on home projects together.
			Step 5

My Maintenance Plan Step 7: Check the current schedules and schedule these outings or projects with my kids. Fear of the kids not wanting to do these new activities. Engage with children to understand their feelings about the planned activities.

Step Seven - Maintenance
Think about the systems you have in place. Are they helping you maintain the processes you have created in Step Five? Tweak whatever is not working as you go.

On a separate piece of paper or use the space below to write out your answers on ways you can ensure you continue with your redesign (new habit). Examples are provided above.

CHAPTER THREE - THE SEVEN WASTES

"The most dangerous kind of waste is the waste we don't recognize."

— SHIGEO SHINGO

This exercise will help you be more specific and accountable to what you set out to do (our new habit). Use your answers from the Seven Adjustment Steps Grid in Chapter Two to re-evaluate your answers with each of the Seven Wastes. You can do this on a separate piece of paper by writing out your answers to the Seven Wastes utilizing your answers from the GRID in Chapter Two. Follow along on the next page(s), using the examples from the Seven Readjustment Steps to understand how you can answer the questions on your waste list.

After reviewing the examples in each activity, begin entering your answers for each waste in the grids on the following pages.

~

1. *What can you improve, eliminate, or redesign?*

Using all your answers from the Seven Readjustment Steps, review and dig deeper and write how you can improve, redesign, or eliminate actions that don't serve you or your goals.

THE SEVEN WASTES

ONE - ACTIVITY

What can you improve, eliminate, or redesign?

Example from Seven Readjustment Steps:

Myself
- No self-care
- Commit to having time to an activity for myself.
- Time constraints. Make "me" a priority. Put it on the calendar.
- Get up 1 hour earlier each morning and meditate.

Example from Seven Readjustment Steps:

My kids
- Too many activities
- Re-evaluate activities
- Fear.
- Engage with children to understand their feelings about the planned activities.
- Add quality time

Examples:
I can improve how I get myself to be consistent in having me time."

Examples:
I can improve on being comfortable with eliminating unnecessary activities.

1.

2.

3.

4.

5.

~

2. How are you getting there?

Using all your answers from the Seven Readjustment Steps, review and dig a little deeper and write how you can find additional ways to get it done.

THE SEVEN WASTES
TWO - CONVEYANCE
How are you getting there?

Example from Seven Readjustment Steps:

Myself
- No self-care
- Commit to having time to an activity for myself.
- Time constraints. Make "me" a priority. Put it on the calendar.
- Get up 1 hour earlier each morning and meditate.

Example from Seven Readjustment Steps:

My kids
- Too many activities
- Re-evaluate activities
- Fear.
- Engage with children to understand their feelings about the planned activities.
- Add quality time

Examples:
> Schedule the "me time" on my phone and share my schedule with my partner. If it requires hiring a sitter, then commit to doing that.

Examples:
> I will create a new activity schedule with my kids' input and limit the number of activities they can do.

1.

2.

3.

4.

5.

~

3. *What is stopping you?*

Using all your answers from the Seven Readjustment Steps, review and explore what is stopping you from getting this accomplished.

THE SEVEN WASTES
THREE - OBSTRUCTION
What is stopping you?

Example from Seven
Readjustment Steps:

Myself
- No self-care
- Commit to having time to
  an activity for myself.
- Time constraints. Make
  "me" a priority. Put it on
  the calendar.
- Get up 1 hour earlier each
  morning and meditate.

Example from Seven
Readjustment Steps:

My kids
- Too many activities
- Re-evaluate activities
- Fear.
- Engage with children to
  understand their feelings
  about the planned
  activities.
- Add quality time

Examples:
  Feeling guilty, excuse of
  no time to do this

Examples:
  Fear that my children will
  be missing out or losing
  an opportunity.

1.

2.

3.

4.

5.

～

4. What appears to be broken in your "everyday" life? How is your quality of life? What are your defects?

Using all your answers from the Seven Readjustment Steps, review and apply these questions to dig deeper for your resolution.

THE SEVEN WASTES
FOUR - SHORTCOMING

What appears to be broken in your "everyday "life?
How is your Quality of Life? What are your defects?

Example from Seven Readjustment Steps:

Myself
- No self-care
- Commit to having time to an activity for myself.
- Time constraints. Make "me" a priority. Put it on the calendar.
- Get up 1 hour earlier each morning and meditate.

Example from Seven Readjustment Steps:

My kids
- Too many activities
- Re-evaluate activities
- Fear.
- Engage with children to understand their feelings about the planned activities.
- Add quality time

Examples:
   Unmotivated, exhausted

Examples:
   Overscheduled, frustration, melt-downs, exhausted

1.

2.

3.

4.

5.

∼

5. Are you overthinking it?

Using all your answers from the Seven Readjustment Steps, review what is relevant to your situation.

THE SEVEN WASTES
FIVE - IRRELEVANT
ARE YOU OVERTHINKING IT?

Example from Seven
Readjustment Steps:

Myself
  - No self-care
  - Commit to having time to
    to an activity for myself.
  - Time constraints. Make
    "me" a priority. Put it on
    the calendar.
  - Get up 1 hour earlier each
    morning and meditate.

Example from Seven
Readjustment Steps:

My kids
  - Too many activities
  - Re-evaluate activities
  - Fear.
  - Engage with children to
    understand their feelings
    about the planned
    activities.
  - Add quality time

Examples:
  Yes, time for myself is
  relevant. Spending time
  trying to justify it is my
  overthinking. There is no
  logical reason why I should
  not spend time on myself.

Examples:
  Creating a cohesive daily
  routine for my children is
  relevant—the thought
  process around what
  everyone else is doing
  needs to be more
  analytical. The focus needs
  to be on what my children are
  interested in and help guide
  them to activities that
  serve them and not others.

1.

2.

3.

4.

5.

~

6. Are you doing too much? Does it bring value?

Review what is excessive using all your answers from the Seven Readjustment Steps. Reevaluate to make sure what you are doing brings value to your life.

THE SEVEN WASTES
SIX - EXCESS
Are you doing too much? Does it bring value?

Example from Seven Readjustment Steps:

Myself
- No self-care
- Commit to having time to an activity for myself.
- Time constraints. Make "me" a priority. Put it on the calendar.
- Get up 1 hour earlier each morning and meditate.

Example from Seven Readjustment Steps:

My kids
- Too many activities
- Re-evaluate activities
- Fear.
- Engage with children to understand their feelings about the planned activities.
- Add quality time

Examples:
I have not spent time on myself. It is something I need to do as it will add value to my daily life and, in return, have a positive impact on my family.

Examples:
Yes. My children are involved in too many activities. They have breakdowns / tantrums, which negatively affect them them and the family. It will be important to begin creating schedules that have them looking forward to the activity. Giving my children a voice in their routine will have a positive impact on them.

1.

2.

3.

4.

5.

~

7. *What do you have or need to get you there?*

Using all your answers from the Seven Readjustment Steps, review and think about what you need to get it accomplished. What are your resources?

THE SEVEN WASTES

SEVEN - RESERVE

What do you have or need to get you there?

Example from Seven Readjustment Steps:

Myself
- No self-care
- Commit to having time to an activity for myself.
- Time constraints. Make "me" a priority. Put it on the calendar.
- Get up 1 hour earlier each morning and meditate.

Example from Seven Readjustment Steps:

My kids
- Too many activities
- Re-evaluate activities
- Fear.
- Engage with children to understand their feelings about the planned activities.
- Add quality time

Examples:
I have made a commitment to my partner and to myself that I should have this time. I schedule the time consistently and get help from family and friends or hire a sitter if necessary. I also have to accept that I am worth it mentally.

Examples:
I have backup plans for who I can utilize to pick up or drop off kids at various activities. My partner, carpooling, family, friends, etc., are good resources for me to use.

1.

2.

3.

4.

5.

CHAPTER THREE - PACT GOALS W/ HABIT

This exercise will help you pick one of your top five Readjustment Steps and create your own PACT goal along with your new habit. Create your PACT Goal below and turn it into a habit. Write the new Cue, Routine and Reward.

Purposeful: These goals are deliberately intended to accomplish what you set out to do.

_____
_____
_____

Actionable: Your plan is ready to go.

_____
_____
_____

Continuous: The action of these goals is continuous and can improve each time.

_____
_____
_____

Trackable: Tracking results will keep you accountable and bring you back to continuous improvements.

_____
_____
_____

New Cue: _____

Routine: _____

Reward: _____

This broad exercise of taking one of your top five from your "Seven Readjustment Steps" and applying it to a PACT Goal illustrates how you can begin to form newer, healthier habits. These new habits can change your life, keep you on track to accomplishing more than you could ever imagine, and feel joy as you move forward.

CHAPTER FOUR- AL-ANON

This exercise will help you dig a little deeper into self-reflection. For each Al-Anon Step, create a statement for yourself to practice. There will be an example statement for each to help you along.

Step 1:

Example: *I am powerless to control everything around me.*

Your statement: _____

Step 2:

Example: *I have faith that everything will work out for the best.*

Your statement: _____

Step 3:

Example: *I will try to let go and not try to control other people's actions.*

Your statement: _____

Step 4:

Example: *I will be honest with myself and take inventory of my daily actions.*

Your statement: _____

Step 5:

Example: *I will think of things I might not be proud of and forgive myself.*

Your statement: _____

Step 6:

Example: *I know I want to change my negative behavior, and I will work hard to find ways to be more positive.*

Your statement: _____

Step 7:

Example: *I will ask for help when needed.*

Your statement: _____

Step 8:

Example: *I will apologize when I do something wrong.*

Your Statement: _____

Step 9:

Example: *I will continue to check in with myself to be sure I am making healthy choices.*

Your Statement: _____

Step 10:

Example: *I will own up to my mistakes and change the behavior if needed.*

Your Statement: _____

Step 11:

Example: *I will try to meditate daily.*

Your Statement: _____

Step 12:

Example: *I will be a mentor to others.*

Your Statement: _____

~

CHAPTER FIVE - AA

This exercise will help you dig deeper into self-reflection and help you let go of what you cannot control. For each Alcoholics Anonymous Step, create a statement for yourself to practice. There is an example statement for each.

Step 1:

Example: *I need to acknowledge that I have no control over my addiction.*

Your Statement: _____

Step 2:

Example: *I will let go of what is bothering me and give it to my higher power.*

Your Statement: _____

Step 3:

Example: *I will try to ask my higher power for help.*

Your Statement: _____

Step 4:

Example: *I will be honest with myself and take inventory of my past behaviors.*

Your Statement: _____

Step 5:

Example: *I will accept the responsibility of doing wrong.*

Your Statement: _____

Step 6:

Example: *I will accept that I need to work on changing my behavior.*

Your Statement: _____

Step 7:

Example: *I will ask for help.*

Your Statement: _____

Step 8:

Example: *I will create a list of people I harmed.*

Your Statement: _____

Step 9:

Example: I will make amends to the people I harmed.

Your Statement: _____

Step 10:

Example: *I will continue to keep an eye on my actions.*

Your Statement: _____

Step 11:

Example: *I will try to meditate or pray daily.*

Your Statement: _____

Step 12:

Example: *I will be a mentor to others.*

Your Statement: _____

~

CHAPTER SIX - LIFE FLOW CHART PROCESS

This exercise will help you get into details in various areas in your life by answering the following questions. You can use information you already have prepared from the earlier chapters to help.

Read through Steps 1 and 2 to familiarize yourself with how your goals should align with your values and beliefs.

1. What are my top five goals?

Are these PACT Goals? [Revisit Chapter 3]

2. Identify what your values and beliefs are.

WHAT IS IMPORTANT TO YOU?

Think about what matters most to you. Is it family? Your health? Is it education and career? Or is it your spirituality, and how do you give back to the community? See if you can pinpoint what drives your beliefs and values. Ask yourself questions like, "*What are my **priorities** in life?*" "*What motivates me?*" "*What do I stand for?*" This can help you to identify what you value the most. Think about where your values and beliefs came from. Have they changed throughout your life?

ANALYZE YOUR EXPERIENCES

Reflect on your life and past experiences, both positive and negative. What did you learn from them? Did you give yourself time to process them? Did you feel the good with the bad? Think about the experiences, people, and events that have shaped your life and have influenced your perspective.

What values and beliefs did you develop from those experiences? Consider what lessons you have learned and what values you hold dear, as this can help you to understand yourself better and clarify your beliefs.

Do my values & beliefs align with my current goals?

Think about your goals. What do you want more of in your life? Thinking about this will help you prioritize the important stuff you want to keep around. Review your top five goals from the previous exercises and see if they align with your values and beliefs.

What do you think your values and beliefs consist of? Think of words that describe what you feel they are or what you want them to be. It may be helpful to break them down into categories or rank them in order of importance. Think about creating a *Value and Belief Statement* reflecting the words you chose to describe them.

Live into your values and beliefs

How will you put your values and beliefs into action? Take a look at your top five goals again and see if these are the actions you need to feel good about what you are trying to accomplish. Use your values and belief system as a guide for making important decisions. As you grow and change, your values and beliefs may also. Be honest and true to your authentic self when defining your values and beliefs and keeping them up-to-date. This is similar to the process of checking your inventory discussed in the 12-step programs.

Try journaling to help you reflect on these thoughts

Make a list of words that might describe what your values and beliefs are.

Can you create a sentence using these words to help you build your values and beliefs? See how many you can come up with.

Do my values and beliefs align with my current goal? Is it simple or complicated? If it is too complicated, re-evaluate

- No. What do I need to readjust?
- Yes. What do I need to re-evaluate?

3. Practice self-reflection. Be mindful of the consequences of your decision-making. Explore your strengths and weaknesses.

What are the consequences of my decision-making (good or bad?), does it reflect my strengths and weaknesses?

When you review your strengths and weaknesses, do you see how they are reflected in your values and beliefs? Will you have positive or negative consequences with your decision or a little of both? Have you thought about what you might be giving up? Remember the economics of your choices. Is it negotiable or black and white? Can you be a little flexible, depending on the situation?

Being mindful of the consequences and what you might be giving up is vital to have successful and positive outcomes. Achieving your goals that align with your values and beliefs will enhance your overall well-being and give you a little joy in your step. Making decisions from emotions and not checking the boxes will most likely give you the negative consequences you are not looking for.

Considering the short and long-term consequences of all your choices is helpful in the decision process.

It's okay to ask for help or find someone you trust to bounce ideas off of. It's healthy to get objective perspectives. Learning to trust others to bring their knowledge and experiences to you is healthy and productive. It is important to try to be open-minded. Feel all the good and the bad in order to learn from these experiences, and find opportunities to help you grow.

DIG DEEPER INTO YOUR STRENGTHS AND WEAKNESSES

1. Think about your personal strengths. What positive, strong character traits come to mind when you think about yourself?
2. Next, write what you know is a weakness. Is this something you can eventually turn into a strength? Review the SWOT Analysis that was introduced to you earlier.
3. Think about your current situation and what opportunities do you think might arise from it?
4. Think about your current situation and what can bring it to failure.

Once you have a better understanding of your strengths, weaknesses, opportunities, and threats in your current situation, you will find the SWOT Analysis to be an amazing tool to use to make decisions more easily.

Of course it is necessary to review as much as you can of what may factor into your decision, depending on the complexity of the decision. A healthy step is to be mindful of all the SWOT and other factors that may influence your outcomes. Go ahead and examine all of it and begin to make informed decisions. Your results will become more mindful and increase your chances of achieving positive outcomes.

Read through **Steps 4 to 6** and focus on self-care and mindset. These steps are continuous.

4. Am I practicing self-care activities?

Am I practicing self-care activities? Reviewing your habits is valuable time spent here.

- What are these activities?
- How often do I practice?

This is an area so many disregard. Taking care of yourself should be a priority. The focus should be on you in a positive manner. Are you prioritizing your self-care activities? Do you leave enough time in the day for you to focus only on you? Doing self-care activities, such as running, painting, meditating, and going out with a good friend are examples of self-care. Remember, it is not selfish to care for yourself. In fact, if you do not take care of yourself it will be difficult for you to take care of others or to get your goals accomplished.

5. Do I let go of negative thoughts and emotions?

LET GO OF NEGATIVE THOUGHTS AND EMOTIONS IN A HEALTHY MANNER

What does this mean? It means it's okay to feel bad when something does not work out or as planned. Feel that emotion. It is also great to feel happy or excited when something good happens. Celebrate! Feel that emotion of success. Sometimes, you can get triggered by something said by someone or even a smell, which can change your mood without you even knowing why or how. This is why it is a good thing to be mindful of how you are feeling and maybe start asking yourself, why?

Whatever the feeling is, accept that you feel a certain way. Try to process it with what you have. You may not always be able to figure it out. Take it in and accept them. Take a deep breath and accept the thoughts and emotions without judgment or criticism. Remember that it's normal to experience negative thoughts and feelings from time to time. It's okay to feel the good with the bad or nothing at all.

When you are feeling negative, and you are in a mood that reflects it, is there a way you can turn it around? Can you change your negative thought process to a positive one? Acknowledge your negative thoughts and then try to simply make positive statements to yourself out loud or, if you need to, in your head. Smile while saying or thinking about them. Look to see if there are any opportunities as many times, if a random change occurs, it does not have to be all bad. By not living in the negative, you may find that your perspective might change a bit when you put a positive spin on it.

Mindfulness Practice: Breathe, breathe, breathe. Being calm and quiet in your own space can be helpful for you to clear your mind, slow down and find the energy to move to your next step. Obviously, being mindful of how you feel or more aware of your emotions can have an influence on how you might be able to change them. Using breathing exercises such as the ones in the previous chapters can also help you to be mindful.

Seek support: Remember your support system is as strong as you allow it to be. Let people in, trust, and learn from these positive forces. If you find it challenging to let go of negative thoughts and emotions, consider seeking support from a trusted friend, family member, or mental health professional. There are so many types of organizations and disciplines out there that are ready to be there for you. Let them! Where or who is in your support system?

Let's remember that it can take practice to accept and let go of negative thoughts or thinking. The more positive you try to be, in practice, the more it may bring us a little more calm and happiness. It does take time, so be kind to yourself. Remember, you matter!

6. Am I practicing gratitude and positive thinking?

PRACTICE GRATITUDE AND BE MINDFUL OF YOUR THOUGHT PROCESS

Are you practicing these habits? Have you created any new habits for you to regularly take time to reflect on what you are grateful for? Do you ever journal your thoughts on what you have gratitude for? It is a good practice to be mindful of what you are grateful for. Focus on what has gone right or even the littlest thing that makes you feel good. Write it down in a book or on paper, just make it convenient for you. I suggest you either do this first thing in the morning so that you have started your day on a good note or in the evening so you can sleep on the great things that happened during the day. Even if it is tiny, write it down.

It takes time, practice, and energy to actively try to reframe negative thoughts into positive ones. Is this a daily practice? Try to make the glass half-full instead of half-empty. Find those positive nuggets in a bad situation or find lessons you might have learned going through the bad experience. Try not to dwell on the negatives, let it go.

It is amazing how good you can make someone else feel when you can express your gratitude to them. *Do you express gratitude towards others?* It's a great feeling when someone thanks you for something or vice versa. It may feel awkward at first, but the more you go out of your way to show gratitude, the easier it will get. You will benefit as well.

Try to find opportunities in situations that don't work out the way you planned. Try to embrace the positivity in the room; if it's not there, bring it. Be with positive, like-minded people. You are who you hang with. Make good choices on who you keep company with.

Do you make an effort to see the good in situations? Instead of dwelling on what went wrong, practicing positivity involves looking for the silver lining in a situation. This is the time to find all of those hidden opportunities to bring you that extra spark of joy!

If you are doing any of the above, you are likely practicing gratitude and positive thinking. Try to do this daily, then try multiple times a day, and you will find yourself improving in all these areas. Remember, there are many resources and practices you can use to cultivate gratitude and positivity in your life. Re-read previous chapters to get that reminder.

How do I do this?

- Journal
- Meditation
- Exercise
- Breathing
- Self-Care Practices

Read through **Step 7**, which goes through the support systems you should have in place. These steps are continuous.

7. Surround yourself with a network of supportive people. Who and what are my resources to help me accomplish my goals?

Who are your go-to people? General suggestions on potential resources that could be helpful in accomplishing your goals.

Personal network: This includes family, friends, colleagues, coaches, mentors. Use your network to support your goals and to provide encouragement when necessary.

Knowledge and skills: Research to find what type of training you might need or special skill sets you want to have. It's in your best interest to keep your skills sharp. What do you have in your toolbox? What can you add?

Tools and technology: The tools and technology available can help you streamline your work and increase your productivity. Seek out what may be helpful and how it will help you get to the next level.

Financial resources: Access to financial resources such as loans, grants, or investors can help you fund your projects and initiatives. Find the right organizations that are willing to give you what you need. Doing the SWOT analysis along with your goal list and the right people will help you figure out what you need to get there.

Time management: Effective time management skills can help you prioritize tasks set deadlines, and manage your workload more efficiently. Creating the habits necessary to manage your day to day will be key here!

Online resources: Social Media, blogs, LinkedIn conversations, online community groups, and even AI applications are great resources to help you find the information you might be looking for or that connection that provides you with the resources you need.

Professional services: Seeking out the right professional service you need is important to help you achieve your goals. Who you need depends on what you are doing. Find the help you need through counselors, coaches, consultants, etc. Don't go with the first one you meet. Make sure it's a good fit with your personality and what you want to get accomplished. Becoming vulnerable is part of the process, and it is important to find someone you can trust.

It's important to identify your specific goals and then evaluate which resources would be most helpful for achieving them. You can also leverage multiple resources to maximize your chances of success. Remember, successful people often surround themselves with the right resources to help them achieve their goals. Again, you are who you hang with. Hang with like-minded people or those with whom you would like to identify.

- Who and what are my resources to help me accomplish my goals?
- Where and who is in your support system? Ask for help!

8. Find professional help when needed. Protect your mental health. Do I find the right help to protect my mental health?

Remember in the previous chapters that it is OKAY to focus on yourself. It is vital for you to take care of yourself! It is necessary to make yourself a priority. This action is not selfish but necessary to grow and feel the joy in your journey. If you are depressed or struggling with your day-to-day life, it is in your best interest to find a therapist, support groups, or other professionals in the mental health arena. You need to make yourself a top priority. It's okay to ask for help.

You no longer need to fake it until you make it. It doesn't need to be that hard. It's okay not to be okay. And when this is your reality, please seek help, as you need to take care of you!

Finally, read through **Step 9 and 10** which help you with continuous improvement along with celebrating your wins.

9. Seek continuous improvement. Find ways to educate yourself and learn as much as you can.

AM I LEARNING AND DEVELOPING NEW SKILLS TO EXPAND
MY KNOWLEDGE AND POTENTIAL?

Revisit where you currently are in your various skill sets and work to learn additional ways to improve on them. It does not have to be everything at once. Pick one at a time. It's gratifying to have continuous improvements in your daily life to help you become your best self. It is a natural process to be curious and seek out more knowledge in the various areas you may have an interest.

Below is a simple list of ways to soak up the information to help you understand and become who you were meant to be. You do you! Don't be afraid! It's never too late!

1. Continuously learn and develop new skills to expand your knowledge and potential.
2. Once you have familiarized yourself with your life flow chart, seek out books or webinars in the areas you want to improve.
3. Am I learning and developing new skills to expand my knowledge and potential?
   o Yes. What are they?
   o No. What can I add?
4. What classes or certifications should you be seeking?

10. Celebrate your wins. Am I celebrating my successes?

Celebrating your successes is important for several reasons:

Boosts Confidence: It just feels good! Simple successes can boost your confidence. It's okay to celebrate a win, even if it is a small one. This can boost your confidence and give you the incentive you need to keep going.
Motivation: When you feel good, your energy will bring on new motivation. Surround yourself with positive, like-minded people to continue the encouragement you need. Having this network will give you the motivation to succeed naturally.
Encourages Progress: Find creative ways to encourage yourself to do more. Maybe add collaborative lunches with key people in your project to bring additional excitement and camaraderie to keep up the good work.

Recognizes Accomplishments: Give yourself little rewards for specific milestones. You will feel proud and continue to strive for your next one. This will keep you striving toward accomplishing even more of those goals. Celebrating these successes is a way of recognizing and acknowledging your accomplishments. It helps you to appreciate how far you have come and what you have achieved, no matter how small or big it is.

Positive Mindset: Keep the positive vibes going. Understand if there are setbacks or some negative outcomes that you find opportunities from this, or take the lessons learned and move on. Find the positives daily to keep that healthy mindset going.

AM I CELEBRATING MY SUCCESSES?

- No. Why not?

Remember, a win is a win. It can be of any size. Focus on what needs to be done and do it in a positive manner, and it will not feel so overwhelming. Bring in the right people to help. Continue to encourage each other and celebrate those accomplishments.

∼

CHAPTER SEVEN - ACCOUNTABILITY CHART

This exercise will help you determine how you are spending your time, and evaluate what changes might be necessary. If you have a worksheet program on your computer, such as Excel, create your own as in the photo on the following page. Otherwise, you can do this on a separate sheet of paper and label it accordingly.

1. Write in **who is doing the task**.
2. Write in the **day of the week** it is being done.
3. Write down the **exact times** each activity is taking.
4. Write **what the task is** and add details to what exactly is happening.

Record your actions for two weeks, from the minute you wake up to the minute you close your eyes. It is a tedious exercise. It is also a very valuable one and will reveal how your time is spent. When I work with my clients in their home, I act as if they are the CEO of their company. Go figure, most of the time, the person that calls me for help is the one doing everything by themselves in the house. So, same thing I tell the CEOs, what can you outsource? What can you stop doing and give it to someone else? Going through this exercise of writing down what you are doing daily will reveal how you are spending your time. You might see patterns and it will be obvious what has to change.

The Accountability Chart will not only help you determine how you are spending your time, but it will also help you evaluate what changes might be necessary. You will have the freedom of a clear understanding of how your time is spent.

Name	Date - Frequency Weekly Daily Hourly M T W Th F Sat Sun	Getting Ready for work	Making breakfast	Making Lunches	Dropping kids off to school	Driving to w…
Who is doing it?	When? Day / Time	Add details to what you are doing?				
Me	Monday 5:00 am	Taking shower/ finding clothes / getting my workstuff together				
Me	Monday 6:30 am		Making me, my partner and kids breakfast			
Me	Monday 7:00 am			Making Lunches for me, my partner and kids		
Me	Monday 7:30 am				Dropping kids to their schools or daycare	

CHAPTER SEVEN - TAPPING

Ready to give it a try? The following tapping sequence is for general stress. Please refer to the tapping points diagram and follow along!

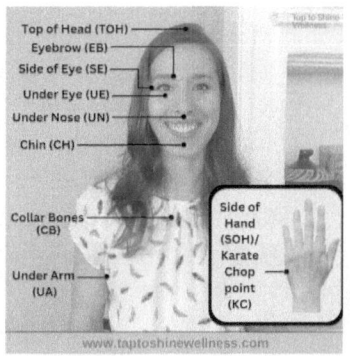

Take a nice easy breath in through your nose and out through your mouth. Start tapping on the side of your hand (SOH), as you read the statements out loud.

SOH: Even though I feel this stress, I accept myself and how I'm feeling right now. Even though I feel this stress in my body, I choose to completely accept myself anyway. Even though I feel this stress, I accept these current feelings, and I love and accept myself anyway.
TOH: This stress
EB: This stress in my body
SE: I'm really feeling it
UE: This stress in my body
UN: All this stress that I'm carrying
CH: I feel so stressed
CB: This heavy stress
UA: This stress in my body
TOH: I accept that I feel this way right now

Take a breath, inhaling through the nose and exhaling slowly through the mouth (like you're blowing out a candle). Take a moment and notice how you feel.

In the next round, replace the word "body" with wherever you feel the stress in your body. If you don't notice any physical sensations, say the phrases as written.

SOH: Even though I have this sensation in my "body" (name where you feel the stress), I love and accept myself anyway.
Even though I feel this stress as a sensation in my "body" (name where you feel the stress), I completely accept myself and how I feel.
Even though I'm feeling this stress as a sensation in my "body" (name where you feel the stress), I completely love and accept myself and all my feelings.
TOH: This stress in my "body" (name where you feel the stress)
EB: This tightness in my "body" (name where you feel the stress)
SE: This stress is showing up as a sensation in my "body" (name where you feel the stress)
UE: What's it telling me?
UN: This stress sensation in my "body" (name where you feel the stress)
CH: Feeling so stressed
CB: And I'm feeling it in my "body" (name where you feel the stress)
UA: This stressful sensation in my "body" (name where you feel the stress)
TOH: This stressful feeling in my "body" (name where you feel the stress)

Take another slow easy breath; inhaling through the nose and exhaling through the mouth. Now, check in with yourself and notice how you feel. Repeat as needed.

Prefer to follow along with a video? You can find the video version of this tapping for stress script on this link:

https://www.youtube.com/watch?v=2jum3q64RXo

Happy Tapping!!

JOYFUL PRACTICE

Chapter Nine - Toolbox Wheel

This exercise should guide you to actions that will improve your daily life. Under each system, begin to review these areas and write down what you can do to work towards your goal.

I will provide six additional sample pieces of the pie (Box Wheel). Now it's your turn to practice. Use the remaining pieces to gain a better understanding of how you can combine the three tool applications to have a more narrow focus on what you need to work on.

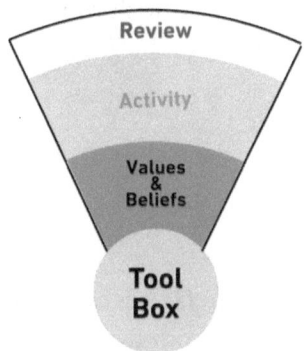

REVIEW

> **Self-Assessment:** Start by reviewing different areas of your life, such as your career, relationships, health, or personal develop-ment. Think about your current situation and identify areas that weigh you down. Begin to see where the need for some improvement is.
> **Reflect:** Think about your current situation and identify areas where you feel dissatisfied.
> **Gather Data:** Collect information related to the areas you're reviewing. Feedback from others or personal observations will help provide you with a good understanding of your current state.

Write down your answers.

ACTIVITY

Goal Setting: Define your life goals and what you want to achieve. Your goals can be in various areas. Choose what is most impactful.

Action Planning: Break down your goals into actionable steps or activities. Make sure your plan outlines the specific tasks and actions you need to accomplish to move closer to achieving your goals and objectives.

Consistency: Implement these activities consistently. Regularly engage in the actions that align with your goals to make meaningful progress over time.

Write down your answers.

VALUES & BELIEFS

Live your values and beliefs: It is essential to live and breathe your values and beliefs. Let's put these values and beliefs into action throughout your daily life. Use them to guide you in all of your decision-making processes. Your values and beliefs can transform through experiences and, over time, evolve into something different. It's important to be vulnerable, honest, and true to your authentic self when diving into your values and beliefs.

Write down your answers.

~

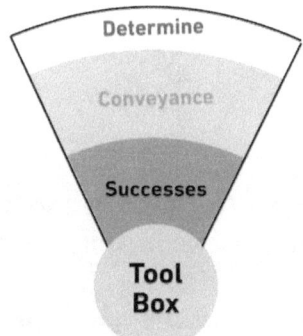

DETERMINE

Set Clear Goals: Determine specific goals and objectives for each area you're looking to improve. Make sure your goals are PACT (Purposeful, Actionable, Continuous and Trackable) to provide clear direction.

Prioritize: Consider the importance and urgency of each goal. Determine which areas require immediate attention and which can be addressed later. This will help you allocate your time and resources effectively.

Write down your answers.

CONVEYANCE

Effective Communication: Focus on improving your communication skills. Effective conveyance of thoughts, ideas, and emotions will enhance your personal and professional relationships.

Listening Skills: Learn to actively listen to others. This skill will help you understand their needs and perspectives, leading to better collaboration and problem-solving.

Clarity: Ensure that your messages are clear and concise. Avoid ambiguity in your communication to prevent misunderstandings and confusion. Be succinct.

Write down your answers.

SUCCESSES

> ***Document Achievements:*** Write down your wins, both big and small. These can be related to your goals or other areas of your life.
>
> ***Celebrate Milestones:*** Celebrate your achievements. Acknowledge your hard work and use your successes as motivation to keep going.

Write down your answers.

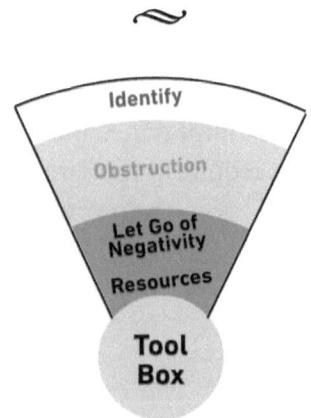

IDENTIFY

> ***Root Causes:*** Identify the underlying causes or obstacles that are preventing you from achieving your goals or living a better life. This step involves a deep analysis of the issues at hand.
>
> ***Strengths and Weaknesses:*** Identify your personal strengths and weaknesses related to the goals you've set. Understand what you excel at and where you need improvement.

Write down your answers.

OBSTRUCTION

Identify Challenges: Look for what might be stopping you from moving forward. This might include external factors or personal limitations.

Problem-Solving: Develop strategies to overcome these obstacles. Consider seeking advice or support from others who have faced similar challenges.

Persistence: Approach obstacles with determination and resilience. Don't let them deter you from pursuing your goals. Instead, view them as opportunities for growth and learning.

Write down your answers.

LET GO OF NEGATIVITY

Identify Negative Influences: Recognize negative people, habits, or situations in your life. Identify what triggers negativity.

Strategies to Let Go: Find what works best to help you let go of negative feelings. Visualize letting go of negative emotions.

Track Progress: Record instances where you successfully let go of negativity and how it improved your overall well-being.

Positive Reinforcement: Surround yourself with positive, like-minded people. Share your successes with supportive friends or family who can provide encouragement.

Self-Compassion: Be kind to yourself. Tell yourself it is okay if you don't make every goal you set. Talk to yourself as if you were talking to a friend.

Write down your answers.

RESOURCES

Financial Management: Create a budget, save, and seek financial advice if necessary.

Time Management: Prioritize tasks, set goals, and delegate when possible. Use tools like planners or apps to manage your time effectively.

Social Resources: Cultivate a supportive social network. Nurture relationships that bring positivity and cut ties with toxic relationships.

Write down your answers.

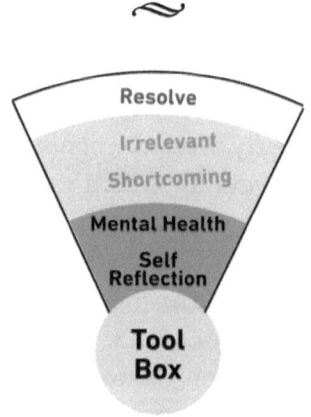

RESOLVE

Problem Solving: Develop solutions and strategies to address the root causes you've identified. Consider different approaches and choose the most appropriate ones for each issue.

Action Plan: Make a detailed list that can help you resolve your problems. Break down your goals into smaller, manageable tasks.

Write down your answers.

IRRELEVANT

Focus on Priorities: Determine what truly matters in your life and prioritize those aspects. Avoid getting distracted or consumed by irrelevant activities or information.

Time Management: Manage your time effectively by dedicating more of it to meaningful tasks toward your goals and less irrelevant tasks or distractions.

Simplify: Declutter your mind and space. Get rid of the things that don't matter to you. This can create more space for what's truly important.

Write down your answers.

SHORTCOMINGS

Self-Awareness: Acknowledge your personal shortcomings and areas where you need improvement. Self-awareness is the first step toward personal growth.

Skill Development: Identify specific skills or qualities that would address your shortcomings. Invest time and effort in developing these skills or improving your weaknesses.

Continuous Learning: Embrace a mindset of continuous learning and improvement. Recognize that everyone has areas where they can grow and evolve.

Write down your answers.

MENTAL HEALTH

Seek Support: Find the mental health professionals you might need to help you.

Practice Mindfulness: Learn mindfulness and meditation techniques.

Monitor Progress: Regularly assess your mental health. Note improvements and setbacks. Adjust your strategies accordingly.

Write down your answers.

SELF-REFLECTION

Identify Patterns: Look for patterns in your successes. What actions or behaviors led to your achievements? Use this information to set strategies for your remaining goals.

Learn from Failures: If you faced setbacks, analyze what went wrong. Learn from your failures. Adjust your approach and try again.

Journaling: Keep a journal to write down your thoughts, emotions, and experiences. Writing can provide insights and emotional release.

Feedback: Seek feedback from trusted friends or mentors. Constructive criticism can help you grow.

Set Personal Goals: Reflect on your values and set goals aligned with them. Regular self-reflection ensures you're on the right path.

Write down your answers.

~

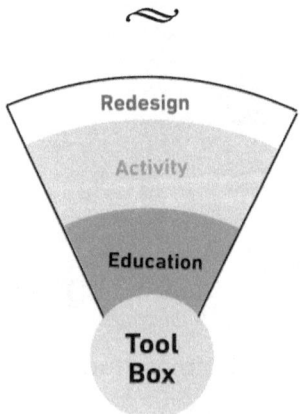

REDESIGN

Process Improvement: Redesign your routines, habits, and processes to align with your goals and solutions. This may involve eliminating inefficiencies or adopting new practices that support your desired outcomes.

Adaptability: Be willing to adapt and change as needed. If your initial approach isn't working, be open to redesigning your strategies for improvement.

Write down your answers.

ACTIVITY

Goal Setting: Begin by defining your life goals and what you want to achieve. These goals can span various areas, such as career, health, relationships, and personal development.

Action Planning: Break down your goals into actionable steps or activities. Create a plan that outlines the specific tasks and actions you need to take to move closer to your objectives.

Write down your answers.

EDUCATION

Learn and Grow: Find ways to learn new skills and give you more knowledge to take on new adventures. Personal growth often leads to new opportunities and successes.

Help Others: As you achieve your goals, consider how you can help others. Sharing your knowledge and resources can create a positive impact on both your life and the lives of others.

Continuous Learning: Find classes, workshops, or special certifications to enhance your skills.

Read Widely: Read books and articles or watch documentaries on diverse topics. Continuous learning broadens your perspective.

Apply Knowledge: Apply what you learn. Knowledge is most valuable when put into practice.

Write down your answers.

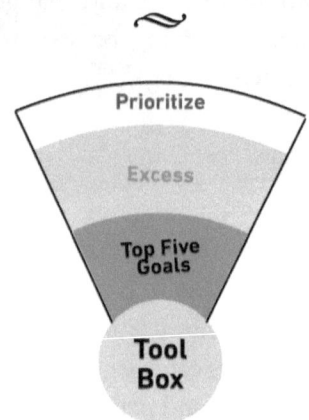

PRIORITIZE

Time Management: Prioritize your tasks and commitments based on their importance and alignment with your goals. This ensures that you allocate your time and energy to what matters most.

Resource Allocation: Be sure to allocate the best resources possible to support your goals. Prioritizing your resources can help you achieve your objectives more efficiently and effectively.

Write down your answers.

EXCESS

Moderation: Moderation, moderation, moderation. No matter what you do in life: food, activities, drinking, buying, etc. all should be done in moderation. It is a healthier approach to daily living.

Minimalism: Life can be simpler by minimizing the material items you may have. You can also apply this to your commitments. Minimizing and simplifying can reduce your stress.

Write down your answers.

TOP FIVE GOALS

Specificity: Clearly define your goals.

Prioritization: Determine which goals are most important to you. Rank your goals from the most important to the least important.

Visualization: Imagine what achieving each goal would look and feel like. Visualization can enhance motivation and focus.

Review and Revise: Regularly review your goals and successes. Your priorities might change, and new opportunities or challenges might arise.

Adjust Goals: If your goals are no longer relevant or if you've outgrown them, don't be afraid to modify them. Your life is dynamic, and your goals should adapt accordingly.

Write down your answers.

∾

Index

CHAPTER FIVE

Letting Go

Letting go is an impressive idea that can change how you look at things in life.

Topics: Physical Clutter; Mental Clutter; Alcoholics Anonymous (AA) 12-Step.

CHAPTER SIX

Making Choices

Take a deeper dive into your values and priorities. You will gain the knowledge on how your choices and decisions should align with your values and beliefs. Utilize the Life FlowChart Process to maintain what you have built.

Topics: SWOT; Life Flow Chart Process.

CHAPTER SEVEN

Set Me Free

Set yourself free and achieve your goals.

Topics: Accountability Chart; Tapping; Sound Baths.

CHAPTER EIGHT

This is It

Think about Joy.

Topics: A Story; Joy.

CHAPTER NINE

You Got This

Focus on the steps that may need extra attention.

Topics: Tool Box Wheel

CHAPTER TEN

Keep it Going

Additional maintenance to keep what you created going

Topics: Checklist (Daily, Weekly, Monthly, Quarterly, Yearly).

CHAPTER ELEVEN

Joyful Practices

Put what you have learned into practice.

Topics: Joy Practice Exercises

Resources

Malepfane, M. (n.d.). *When life happens*. PoemHunter. https://www.poemhunter.com/poem/when-life-happens/

Maslow's hierarchy of needs (a complete guide). (2022, December 8). *OptimistMinds*. https://optimistminds.com/maslows-hierarchy-of-needs/

Maslow's hierarchy of needs. (2023, June 8). *Simply Psychology*. https://www.simplypsychology.org/maslow.html

Maslow, A. H. (1943). *A theory of human motivation*. Psychological Review, 50(4), 370-396. https://doi.org/10.1037/h0054346

Hughes, L. (n.d.). *She, within herself, found loveliness....* Goodreads. Retrieved November 24, 2024, from https://www.goodreads.com/quotes/9762897-she-in-the-dark-found-light-brighter-than-many-ever

Lean manufacturing. (n.d.). *Wikipedia*. https://en.wikipedia.org/wiki/Lean_manufacturing
Law, J. (Ed.). (2009). *A Dictionary of Business and Management*. Oxford University Press.

Emad, S. (2017, May 23). The most dangerous kind of waste is the waste we do not recognize. *LinkedIn*. https://www.linkedin.com/pulse/most-dangerous-kind-waste-we-do-recognize-shigeo-emad

Duhigg, C. (2018, February 2). *Notes on The Power of Habit*. Medium. https://medium.com/@aidanhornsby/notes-on-the-power-of-habit-8d8b93df8069

Clear, J. (2018, March 7). Warren Buffett's "2 List" strategy: How to maximize your focus and productivity. *James Clear*. https://jamesclear.com/buffett-focus

Helmsley, B. **Talking to the Wild**. (2021). *She sat at the back and they said she was shy. She led from the front and they had no words*. In *Talking to the Wild: The bedtime stories we never knew we needed*. Wildmark Publishing.

Al-Anon Family Groups. (n.d.). *Welcome to Al-Anon Family Groups*. Retrieved November 24, 2024, from https://al-anon.org/

Evoke Waltham. (n.d.). *The 12 steps of Al-Anon: A framework for addiction recovery*.

Evoke Waltham. Retrieved December 3, 2024, from https://www.evokewaltham.-com/rehab-blog/the-12-steps-of-al-anon-a-framework-for-addiction-recovery/

Niebuhr, R. (n.d.). *The Serenity Prayer* (Unabridged version)

Alcoholics Anonymous. (n.d.). *The twelve steps of Alcoholics Anonymous*. Retrieved November 24, 2024, from https://www.aa.org/the-twelve-steps

Owls Nest Recovery. (n.d.). *What are the 12 steps of AA?* Owls Nest Recovery. Retrieved December 3, 2024, from https://www.owlsnestrecovery.com/blog/what-are-the-12-steps-of-aa

Visual Thesaurus. (n.d.). *Synonym for "sorrow", "joy"*. Retrieved November 24, 2024, from https://www.visualthesaurus.com/app/view

McMillan, G. (n.d.). *You've got this*. Cosmofunnel. Retrieved November 24, 2024, from https://cosmofunnel.com/poems/youve-got-this-156690

Wilcox, E. W. (n.d.). *I am*. Your Daily Poem. Retrieved November 24, 2024, from https://www.yourdailypoem.com/listpoem.jsp?poem_id=4176

Dyson, S. (2021). *Follow me on this*. Red Thread Publishing. (Dyson, 2021, p. 45)

FLOW

(FOR JACQUELINE HILL)

Girl
you got this

you got this
Voice
begging to be borne on the wind
needing to be out defining new parameters and making
magic

you got this Will
that time and tears have attempted to break
(you can't be broken)
that's been trampled like a diamond in the dust
pick it up, dust it off
start a fire from all the thousand shining facets

You don't wait on easy
or convenient
or if/ when/ wonder
you run
you fly
Now
you sing
Loud
and if they can't keep pace
that's too bad
but you don't fold your wings and drag feet
for a
ny
body

Folks better pray up and come on
'cause you got this
this insistent ringing in your heart
from the ancestors
urging/demanding
you tell your story the best way you know
the only way it can be told
with heart
with honor
with an ineffable sense of being

with love

And a lot of folks won't like it
won't care
can't get it
that is not your concern
you may pity them (Girl, you don't have that kind of time)
you may scorn (Girl, you don't have that kind of heart)

You can only do service to the world
by being faithful with yourself
true with yourself

sing the songs honestly
don't you shape those notes for safety
shape them for celebration
shape them for risk
shape them for prophecy

Folks better just pray up
get right and hold on

'Cause, Girl
you got this

this vision
Run paint the sky and the wind with words

NO thing NO body
can destroy/ignore/alter/deny

and step sweet and look good while you do it
('cause you know that's how we roll)

Pain?
oh yes
Doubt?
believe it

Insecure confusions?
yes indeed
all those right there

Nights when fear makes your mind freeze
days when the words mock you from a haven
just beyond the reach of your fingertips
when Frustration nags at you like a bitter old auntie
who has no friends and your cellphone number

Breathe
Pray
Dance
Eat dark chocolate with almonds

Make love
whatever it takes, whatever works
to remind you that denial of your tales and talent
is not known in the grand scheme of things

You can get weary
but don't get lost
You can get mad/crazy/disgusted
but you don't quit/get lazy/lose focus
or fire

Breathe
Love
take it al-l-l-l-l
in stride
and step sweet and look good while you're doing it
'cause you know that's how we roll

Girl
You
GOT
this

This way to redefine the world
and the words

Sing
Risk
run with all of it

FLY
and never forget the way and will
of the thousands women before
the way and will of the five thousands coming
are sweetening the road beneath your feet
and the wind at your back
all of us praying/crying/ cheering you forward
praying/ singing/ shouting one single, sacred phrase
"Go, just go
just go
ON"

'Cause, Girl
You got this.

Dyson, S. (2021). *Follow me on this*. Red Thread Publishing.

About the Author

Rosetta grew up in Chicago, married and has three children. She is a Professional Organizer, System's Strategist and a Joyologist, passionate about helping people navigate their dreams, disappointments, and realities to find peace of mind. With extensive experience as a System Strategist and Lean Six Sigma Black Belt certified professional, she excels in identifying opportunities for continuous improvement in both personal and professional spaces.

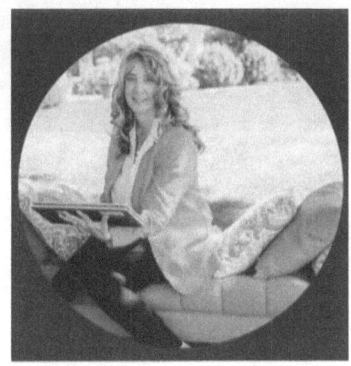

Photo Credit Lisa Kay Photography

She has a natural knack for organization. In 2016, Rosetta debuted her organizing business, Lettuce Organize. As the Founder, Rosetta has established a recognized service in the Chicagoland area, specializing in the home and workplace. Her expertise in organizational assessment, planning, workflow analysis, process mapping, decluttering, and staging, all aimed at fostering a healthier lifestyle.

Rosetta has always been community-oriented. When you grow up in a household of 13 people, you get used to being around others and helping along the way. It's in her DNA.

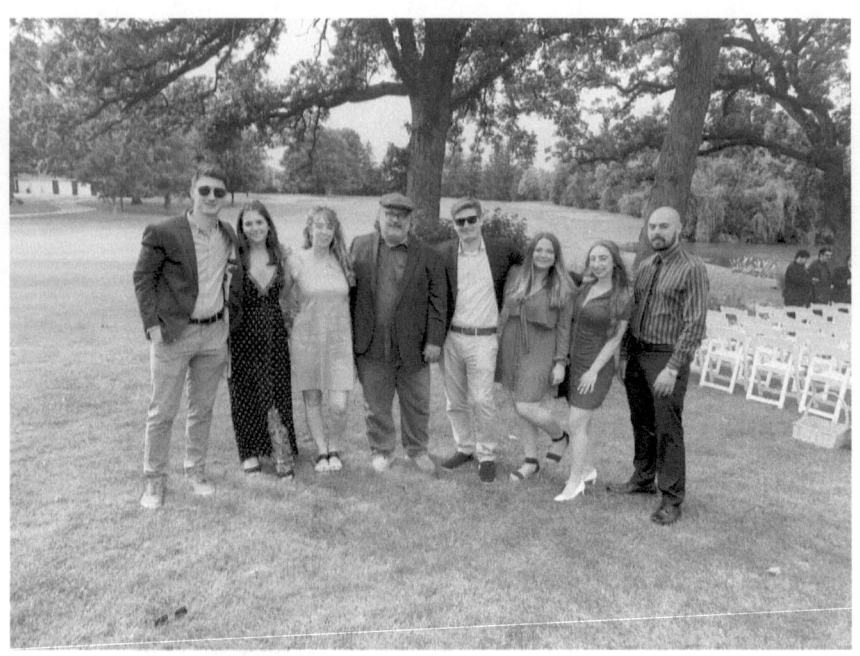

Through all of life's ups and downs, Rosetta has realized that you must find joy in the journey. That you have the power to reflect, discover what drives you, and create a roadmap to reach your goals joyfully. To learn more about Lettuce Organize, go to https://linktr.ee/info219.

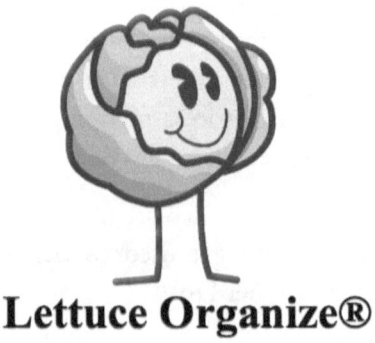

Lettuce Organize®

**Lettuce Organize your tomorrow
so you can enjoy today. SM**

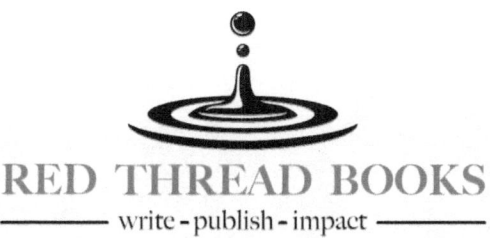

RED THREAD BOOKS

———— write - publish - impact ————

Publish with Red Thread Books, an imprint of Red Thread Publishing.

We provide expert guidance to nonfiction authors through every stage of the publishing process. Visit **www.redthreadbooks.com** to learn more and connect with our team.

REVIEW THIS BOOK

Enjoyed *The Joy Journey*? Your feedback means the world! If the book resonated with you, inspired you, or offered something meaningful, we'd truly appreciate it if you left a review. Your feedback helps others discover the book—and it directly supports the author's work.

www.ingramcontent.com/pod-product-compliance
Lightning Source LLC
Chambersburg PA
CBHW021639120626
46545CB00002B/621